MW01295332

Sudden Intimacies

DR. JIM DAVIS MD

435 770 1234
2189 Chippeham Ct
StG   84770

Copyright © 2021 Dr. Jim Davis MD
All rights reserved
First Edition

PAGE PUBLISHING, INC.
Conneaut Lake, PA

First originally published by Page Publishing 2021

ISBN 978-1-6624-1529-6 (pbk)
ISBN 978-1-6624-1530-2 (digital)

Printed in the United States of America

Dedicated to Cathy Davis for being there with me all
these years and experiencing all that life has to offer, as
well as listening to countless retellings of these stories.

Special thank you to Amy Davis and Tom Davis
for helping bring this book to print.

A special thank you to Callie Reagan for her insights and edits.

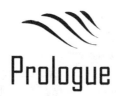

Prologue

Through my whole professional career, I have known that physicians were to be considered as trusted individuals. We share with them a variety of secrets and information that we generally don't entrust with others, including, at times, our spouses or others closest to us. I always thought it curious that we would, in many different circumstances, trust relatively complete strangers with this information. As I learned more and more through my careers in family medicine and emergency medicine, I became aware of a characteristic of the private doctor's office or emergency department (ED) encounter that was really quite unusual and powerful. It occurred to me once while I was contemplating issues surrounding patient care that patients really relegated to me quite a bit of authority and power over many aspects of their personal lives, their privacy, and their bodies. What I noticed was that I could enter a room with someone even a total stranger and the Aesculapian authority (named after Aesculapius, the Greco-Roman god of medicine) conferred on me by my job as a physician allowed me certain privileges with the patient or family members. Now I realized almost immediately that with this authority and power came a tremendous responsibility.

This power would enable me to ask very personal and even embarrassing questions—such as, about a history of drug abuse, what their deepest medical concerns and fears were, what their family history entailed, even such personal questions as whether or not they were faithful to their spouse, were concerned about STIs, fears about heart disease, concerns about diet, and many other very personal and otherwise taboo topics.

I found that most patients would readily permit me to explore these areas of fears, hopes, dreams, and personal issues, almost without question. In addition to that, they would permit me, in fact, they would expect that I would examine their bodies closely in a most personal fashion without risk of concerns for their safety, exposure, or previous unfamiliarity with me as a person. This process of opening themselves completely to a stranger I called "sudden intimacies" is a characteristic of most aspects of medicine but is particularly strong in the realm of emergency medicine where patients routinely submit themselves to evaluation, painful or inconvenient testing, as well as to uncomfortable or even frightening treatments. These experiences are carried out on a daily basis in every emergency room in the country. The emergency physician must balance these allowed latitudes on the patient's behalf with a trust and commitment to maintain the patient's confidence and only do those things, which are both necessary and in the patient's best interest. In order to properly use this power offered to emergency physicians, one had best present themselves as professional in both action and dress and attempt at all times to maintain the confidence that what is being requested is in the patient's own best interest. Any breach of this mutual contract can result in the patient declining further care, refusal of further services, and even concerns over malpractice. Balancing the power offered to the clinician by such patients as present to emergency departments with the responsibility to always act in the patient's best interest and recalled the historic Latin phrase *primum non nocere*, which translates to "first, do no harm." This implied two-way contract between the clinician and the patient is how successful modern medicine operates.

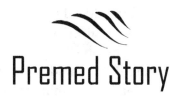

Premed Story

From the time of my late teenage years when I became serious about my future career, I knew I wanted to be a chemist. Looking back on this, it was really an unrealistic plan implemented because my older brother was a chemist and I liked chemistry as a high school subject and had adopted a high school chemistry teacher as my favorite teacher. Despite this, I frequently entered science fair projects into regional and statewide competitions in the area of biological projects and failed to recognize this tendency, preferring instead, to look at my brother's career with envy because of my respect for him. As a result, I chose a college that offered an ACS certification in chemistry. I also chose to play college football and received a scholarship offer at a school in western Illinois, not far from my hometown. The key points to making this decision included my desire to stay with a smaller school rather than a large university owing to potential class size and my comfort level, having grown up in rural Iowa. I also chose chemistry although I was offered a scholarship to study physics during my senior year in high school. I went off to school that fall of my freshman year in college thinking that I would become a chemist, perhaps teach, or otherwise enter the industry in some capacity. Along the way, several things happened to change my plans.

During fall of my sophomore year, one of my chemistry professors came to class and asked the question, "How many of you are chemistry majors?" He then proceeded to display the back cover of a weekly magazine entitled *Life*, which contained numerous photographs of current news events—at that time, mostly about the Vietnam War. The inside cover in the back was a recurrent photo essay entitled "Parting Shots," which tried to tell a story using a single photograph to make its point. That particular week's photograph was of a young man standing in a laboratory setting, wearing a white laboratory jacket, and carried the title "Doesn't Anybody Need a PhD Chemist?" The photograph contained several curious sheets of paper hanging from the ceiling of the laboratory. The story represented the situation faced by a young PhD candidate, ready to graduate, who was having difficulty finding work within the field of chemistry. My professor's point was that jobs were difficult to find within the field, and those of us who were chemistry majors might want to rethink our position.

I went up after class and studied the photograph carefully thinking to myself that I had better make a change in plans. I spent the remainder of that day discussing this with my girlfriend, who was later to become my wife, asking her opinion about how this might affect my future. I also contacted my brother, the chemist, who reported that there were, indeed, no jobs of any significant number available in the field of chemical research, teaching of chemistry, or the industry. Based on this discussion, my girlfriend asked me if I'd ever thought about medicine as a career, stating that my father had always made comments about me becoming a physician, which was a dream that he had quietly held for some time. I gave this some deep thought, coming to the realization that my interests were really more aligned with medicine than chemistry and that I knew I would be comfortable in any field so long as it were scientific in nature and involved measuring, weighing, and decision-making based on scientific principles. This resulted in me eventually being able to provide help, knowledge, and interaction with others. Medicine was, it turned out, the perfect choice for me. Most of my friends were, at the time, premed majors, so it was easy for me to seek advice to find a direct path into that profession.

My plans soon evolved into changing schools from the small private college to the University of Iowa to pursue premedical studies, marrying the girlfriend, moving to Iowa City, and giving up my football scholarship. This plan also involved supplementing my acquired chemistry knowledge with a more rounded science background, including additional biology, physics, and math. For example, I'd had introductory biology but no advanced courses. I had not had introductory physics and needed to add that to my curriculum. In addition, I finished the courses I needed for my chemistry major credit. I even had time left over for an elective class or two in my fourth year. I was able to combine some of the required classes with broader topics that were of interest to me, and so I really wasted no credits on the transfer process. For example, at the university, I was able to take astronomy from Dr. James A. Van Allen as one of my physics credits and loved the experience. I was also able to combine the requirement for additional biology courses with the class in nursing physiology offered by the college of nursing. I ended up losing no time from school and graduated having taken the medical college admissions test and rounded out my education. Several significant events occurred as a result of this decision to transfer to the University of Iowa, which later played important roles in my practice, hobbies, teaching, and life.

The transfer to the University of Iowa created a lot of new circumstance in my life. It was a much larger school, and now that I was married, I was essentially starting over with a new life. Additionally, I was planning on being more self-reliant, and therefore upon moving to Iowa City, immediately found a couple of jobs working hourly. One job was as a dishwasher for a local restaurant named Mr. Steak. There was nothing glamorous about this job, but it helped pay the bills. In order to supplement my income further, I began working at a local service station on weekends while getting ready to attend the university. I was working at these two jobs, not enjoying life very much, when an acquaintance informed me of the potential availability of a new job with a professor at the university who was asking for someone who had chemistry background. I went into the job interview without really knowing much about what was being requested, but I had confidence in my ability to work around chemicals and to do research. I had spent the previous Christmas working through vacation in the college laboratory, having obtained a National Science Foundation grant in the area of inorganic chemistry.

The professor's laboratory was located in the brand-new Basic Sciences Building at the University of Iowa. There I met, for the first time, a professor whom I will call as Dr. T. Now he was a member of the staff of the anatomy department, in the college of medicine, and he was looking for someone for his laboratory who could prepare solutions of various concentrations to help them in his research. His area of research involved microscopic anatomy and the study of various types of muscles. In particular, he was looking at what happens to muscles when they hypertrophy—which is, either through exercise or some other stimulus, when the muscle is induced to become larger and stronger. This was relevant for a variety of reasons because it is the method by which muscles get larger with exercise, get smaller when injured, or in the case of the heart, when a greater load is placed on it by high blood pressure. He was using a variety of models to look at the process of hypertrophy in both skeletal muscle and cardiac muscle. He used various staining techniques and other methods of assay as well as electron microscopy to examine the changes that occurred in the muscle under various stimuli.

Admittedly, I didn't, at that time, know much about any of these topics, but I knew that I was very interested in securing the job. His interview with me consisted of a series of questions related to the mixing of solutions of various concentrations. For me, it was very easy, having just finished a semester of preparing solutions as a teaching assistant for all the classes held at the college I had been attending. His toughest question to me was, having a solution of a given concentration, how much the solution must be diluted by water to achieve a solution of a new concentration. Now this process is very easy, once learned for the first time. He asked, "If I have a solution of 70% alcohol, how much do I dilute to make it 35% alcohol?" The answer to this involves using a graduated cylinder and, in this situation, filling it up to the line marked 35 with a more concentrated alcohol and then diluting it to the line marked 70 with water. He asked me a couple of times using other dilutions at which time he realized how simple the process really was. As a verbal test of my knowledge of the procedure, he gave me the same problem using 100% alcohol and diluting it to 70% alcohol. My response was to fill the graduated cylinder up to the line that indicated 70 mL using the concentrated alcohol and then fill it with water up to the line that indicated 100 mL. He realized that this checked out correctly. At that point, he said, "Is it all that easy?" I replied, "Yes, it's that easy!"

He smiled at me thoughtfully and then said, "Well, I don't think I'll need your help anymore, but because you know how to do that, I think you would be very valuable in my laboratory." That was the beginning of a working relationship with Dr. T. that lasted through the rest of my undergraduate years and onto the first two and half years of medical school, where I continuously worked for him, in his laboratory, part-time while going to school. This job, in addition to being extremely relevant to my future study of medicine, assisted me in receiving his strong recommendation when it came time for my application to medical school as well as generating enough income with this one job that I was able to give up the other two entirely.

As I became more deeply involved in his research, he taught me the processes and techniques of preparation of slides for light microscopy as well as the preparation of tissues for electron microscopy. From this experience, which involved the daily production of sixty to seventy black-and-white 8 × 10 photographs, I also learned much about photography and picked up amateur photography as a hobby. Moreover, over the next several years, I participated actively in his research as a research assistant and had my name added to several publications that appeared in professional anatomy journals. Of course, none of this looked bad nor hurt me on my application to medical school when the time for that arrived.

Part of the research that he was doing involved the ultrastructure of cardiac muscle in its response to the load placed upon it by rising blood pressure. The model that we used was most commonly a strain of white rat, which spontaneously develop hypertension around four to six weeks of age, which caused changes that we were trying to track to see whether or not when cardiac muscle hypertrophies, does it do so by increasing the number of fibers of muscle tissue present, or does it accomplish the hypertrophy by increasing the size (diameter) of each individual fiber. This information, as I've mentioned, was directly related to human illness in a variety of forms and was of particular interest not only in heart disease but also in the area of exercise physiology, such as running marathons. The changes we were looking for in both skeletal and cardiac muscle were related to the amount of glycogen stored, the number of mitochondria present (see it's directly related to energy metabolism), and the size of the bundles of muscle fiber present within the muscle.

By the time I started my first day of medical school, I was already well acquainted with most of the faculty of the departments of anatomy, exercise physiology, and cardiology. Additionally, I was published and had a good knowledge of what was required to prepare manuscripts for publication in professional journals. I had also taken and passed the medical school class in histology, so I didn't have to retake it during my freshman year, rather I served as a teaching assistant for my fellow classmates during that part of the semester.

Notable Undergraduate Classes

I took many classes as an undergraduate, which made an impression on me, obviously, but perhaps none more than when I took astronomy at the University of Iowa. Now Iowa, at the time, had an astronomer named James A. Van Allen, who served as the department chair and taught several courses, including an introductory course in astronomy. Of course, I learned a lot of basic astronomy, which led me to a lifelong interest in the topic, and I vowed that if I ever lived in an area with dark skies and had sufficient funding, I would own a telescope. (I now own seven telescopes.)

During the course of that introductory class, I was required to complete an assignment by creating an example of astrophotography. I chose for my project to create a montage of the moon as seen from the earth. I chose this topic because this was the mid-seventies and in the prime of the Apollo project, which resulted in humans visiting the moon on several different occasions. I thought I would map the landing sites for my own interest, and later, my laboratory assistant persuaded me to create a large four-foot version of this map to display to the public in the entry foyer of the physics building.

In order to complete this project, I had to obtain several photographs of the visible portion of the moon on several subsequent nights. The reason for this is—due to the natural motion of the moon and its relative position to the earth—the appearance of the moon changes nightly. On any given night, more or less of the moon is visible from the surface of the earth. In addition, the orbits of the earth and moon vary in distance from each other, causing the size of the image visible through a telescope to change by a small amount daily. In order to have the photographs line up properly, I needed to obtain several different examples from which to choose. This resulted in my scheduling a visit to the observatory, located atop the seven-story physics building in downtown Iowa city from where I would make the observations. This building, although located in mid-downtown Iowa City, was tall enough that there was not much light pollution visible to impair the photographic process. All I had to worry about was weather, particularly intervening clouds, and my schedule.

I obtained the proper clearance from the graduate assistant in charge of the class and scheduled my observing nights. There were specific instructions with regards to the use of the six-inch refractor telescope mounted in the dome observatory atop that building. As it was a very expensive instrument and was used by many graduate students, I was always careful to use it in accordance with the rules, taking proper care to always point it at zenith (straight up) when I finished my observing in order to prevent dust or moisture from collecting in the telescope. After a few nights of observing and collecting photographs, I came to the observatory one night at about dusk and found the door locked as usual, but the telescope was pointed horizontally with the dome closed. This was unusual in that it was supposed to be pointed straight up, not horizontally, and I thought that I perhaps had left it in the wrong position since I was one of the few students using the instrument at that time. That night, when I finished observing, I dutifully pointed it straight up, put the dust-cover in place, and closed the observatory prior to leaving for home. The following night, I returned again about dusk only to find the telescope once again pointed at the horizon and thought that I might get blamed for the improper storage position of the telescope, and so I mentioned it that evening to the graduate student on duty. He smiled but didn't say anything.

The next time I came to the observatory, I once again found the telescope at the horizontal position and vowed to set the record straight with the graduate student in charge to be certain that I was not blamed for the improper storage position of that telescope. When I reported to him that I found the telescope oriented horizontally, he just smiled and said, "Yes, did you bother to look through it?" I indicated that I had not; to which he said, "Well, you probably should look through it." I went back to the dome atop the roof, entered the observatory, and looked through the uncovered telescope. That expensive, high-quality six-inch optical instrument was pointed squarely at the tenth floor of the girls' dormitory building several blocks away! I became aware of a couple of important teaching points from that experience. First, astronomical telescopes provide an inverted image, which means that everything that you see is upside down. That apparently didn't bother the grad students, who would sneak up in the afternoons to use the telescope for surreptitious purposes. The second thing that I learned from that experience was that astronomy grad students were obviously interested in heavenly bodies of various types, not just the astronomical ones!

South Dakota University Interview

At the time of my application to medical school, I was a senior in my undergraduate program at the University of Iowa. I remember anxiously watching the mail on a daily basis for any letters originating at the schools to which I had applied. My main interest, of course, was the University of Iowa, which was my state school, and would have provided much lower tuition, but I was willing to entertain any school that would give me an offer. Toward the end of the application cycle, I received a letter from my first successful interview requests. The school making the offer was University of South Dakota, in Vermillion, South Dakota. I immediately telephoned them and set up my interview with them. This wasn't the first time I'd ever been to South Dakota because my parents had taken me to Mount Rushmore on a family vacation during my earlier years.

This was my first interview for professional school, and I really didn't know what to expect, but with great apprehension, I made hotel reservations and traveled with my father to Vermillion, South Dakota. On the night prior to my interview, we arrived in a fairly small town of Vermillion, and I had to admit that I was less than impressed. The University of South Dakota was a newly formed four-year school, which provided basic science education for the first two years on the Vermillion campus and then transferred its students to the University of Minnesota for their clinical rotations. While this program, at first, appeared less than optimum, I was interested in them because they were interested in me. The town of Vermillion, as I mentioned, was very small with very few opportunities for shopping, the major provider being a Sears catalog store. Admittedly, the university was easy to navigate, and I readily found the administration building during my drive around that night. I was very apprehensive and didn't sleep well through the night in anticipation of my interview the following morning. Of course, I wore a suit and tie and put on my best manners, in addition to my best dress and drove over with my father to the university's administration building where the interview would occur. I remember being impressed by the friendliness of the staff while introducing myself to the program secretary.

At the appointed time, I was led into a room with a large rectangular table and was seated at the very end of the table, with my back to the windows. A six-member interview team filed in very solemnly and introduced themselves. There were two medical students, one administrator, and three physicians. After exchanging pleasantries about my travel and some small talk aimed at reducing my anxiety, they began rounds of questioning. Each of the interviewers apparently had a copy of my university transcript in their hand and referred to it frequently during the questioning. Probably because it was traumatically memorialized in my long-term memory, the process remains clear to me to this day, and I frequently referred to it when discussing interview processes with premedical students at Utah State University.

The process used by the interviewers consisted of asking first a very general question, such as What kinds of things do you like to do? After hearing my response to this general question, the question was then asked again seeking more detail, such as What kind of music do you like? Do you listen to anything other than popular music? And in a more specific question, such as What is the last classical piece that you heard performed? At the time, I didn't recognize it, but this had been the pattern that was to be repeated over and over throughout the interview process. A very general question was asked focusing my attention on a topic, followed by a more specific question seeking more detail, followed by an even more specific question seeking further detail, followed by a very specific question seeking to flesh out actual details in my level of knowledge regarding the subject. An example of this was the question I see from your transcript that you had biochemistry. What did you find interesting in the area of biochemistry?

My response to this was "I thought the Krebs cycle was very interesting within biochemistry."

To which, the follow-up question was this, What specifically about the Krebs cycle did you find interesting?

My response was "I found the exquisite control points in various parts of the Krebs cycle to be very interesting."

This was followed by these questions, What are some of the specific control points within the Krebs cycle? Can you name them?

I knew several of these control points and, in fact, had recently taken my final exam on the Krebs cycle and could recite it from glucose all the way to carbon dioxide and water along with each of the control points. I talked specifically about the cytochrome system in the mitochondria and how the various chemical processes were controlled both by limits placed on the reactants, the various energies required to drive the mitochondrial respiratory system, and the limitations produced by buildup of products of respiration. This line of questioning only ended when I finally reached the limit of my knowledge and had to answer that I didn't know the exact control of one of the mitochondrial systems.

A couple of other examples readily came to mind. One inquisitor asked, "I see that you've just taken astronomy from Dr. James Van Allen, this spring. I've often wondered, What are the Van Allen belts? I had indeed just taken this course but had not yet taken my final exam and was all studied up on the topic. I told him that the Van Allen belts are collections of particles that carry an electrical charge and orbit around the poles of the earth traveling through space, oscillating between the two poles. Curious, he asked the follow-up question, "What is the period of oscillation of a particle in the Van Allen belts?" Now I assure you that I remembered the answer at that time, but no longer could recall that bit of information now.

Another examiner quizzed me about my exposure to classical music beginning with the open-ended question, "What kind of music do you like?" I replied, "Classical music, mostly," and that response was mostly due to the influence of my wife, who admired and listen to classical music all the time. The first follow-up question asked me to expound on that by listing the most recent classical pieces that I'd listen to, and as it happened, I had tickets that spring to the concert series at the University of Iowa concert center, located along the Iowa River. They further quizzed me as to which performers I had recently heard and what pieces they had performed. This was followed by the question that ultimately showed the limit of my knowledge. "How many symphonies did Beethoven write?" My feeble answer was "a lot. I know he wrote at least nine." The examiner smiled as I had reached the limit of my knowledge and I vowed to look up the answer later on.

This manner of questioning was repeated several times over the next hour. I was asked questions as diverse as Who is playing today for the NBA championship? In the past six weeks, eight Western countries have had shakeups or turnovers in their government, can you name them? What is the predominant color in the painting *The Scream*? and other similar though very specific questions. Each of these questioning lines began as a very general question to orient me to the topic. The questions were very penetrating and covered a wide variety of topics. It was only after talking with many other students about their interview process that I finally determined the reason behind their penetrating questions. Not only were they interested in me as a student wanting to see how full my body of knowledge was with regards to my studies but also looking specifically at my retention and my aptitude for well-rounded topics.

I heard of other students in similar situations were placed in a room with a single window that was painted shut and sometime during the course of the interview, they were asked to stand, turn around, and open the window for fresh air. This, of course, was an impossible task, as was presumably my test of general knowledge to the depth that they were exploring. The purpose of this, of course, was not really to test my level of knowledge, but rather to see how I reacted in a stressful situation. I subsequently realized that the breadth of knowledge required by even basic physicians is extreme. Additionally, the initial level of knowledge must be constantly added upon through continuing education to be certain that it remains current and correct. Simply there is far too much to know so that the practitioner cannot know everything, cannot be expected to learn everything, and certainly cannot be expected to remember everything. The challenge then becomes how does a clinician's behavior or personality change when they are confronted with the limit of their knowledge? Do they fall into a crumbling mass, make up a false answer, or do they simply say, "I don't know?" and proceed on with whatever step is next. This was the process to which I was subjected to at this interview, penetrating to the depth of my knowledge until I no longer knew the answer to the question in order, I believe, to test my durability under stress.

The interview process was followed a week later by a letter of acceptance from the University of South Dakota College of Medicine. I was, at that time, on the alternate list waiting for a position to open at the University of Iowa, and when that opportunity arose, I gratefully seized it and called the University of South Dakota to see under what circumstances I could receive a refund of my deposit and cancel my registration. The friendly voice of that same secretarial staff person greeted my question with "Why, Jim did the University of Iowa accept you?" I readily told her that they did, and she said, "That's wonderful. We'll get your money right back to you."

The University of South Dakota had subsequently became a full-time four-year school, but because of the difference in cost between in-state and out-of-state tuition, I was certainly grateful for the opportunity I had to attend the University of Iowa.

Emerson-Goodwin's Syndrome

After all the ups and downs and preparation and fear, time finally passes by enough to bring about the first day of medical school. As the day arrives, you realize that everything you have done so far has been directed at getting you to this point. With any luck, somebody sends you out the door, off for your first day of classes.

I entered the outer doors of the gross anatomy lab with several of my classmates. A few steps ahead were the inner doors. I could already detect the odor of the preservation fluids that are used to keep the donated bodies from spoiling. I wasn't afraid of the bodies. I had been around recently deceased persons quite often during my younger years. I had witnessed many autopsies in my early and mid teens. My father was employed as a pathology tech. As such, he prepared the recently deceased patients for their postmortem examination and assisted the pathologist in performing the exposure, collection, and evaluation of medical specimen tissues during the autopsy exam. The process of learning gross anatomy was going to be similar. We would be expected to dissect, expose, identify, label, and memorize all the important structures of the body. I had a pretty clear idea of the quantity of information that I'd needed to commit to memory, along with all the other coursework that I'd be doing. I wasn't afraid of facing death, and I wasn't going to be *grossed out* by the cadaver lab. I just knew the challenge before me and was only intimidated due to the volume of learning that I would face.

I entered the second set of doors and saw, for the first time, the vast area of the anatomy lab. There were over one hundred tables, each containing a black-zippered body bag, with the vague shape of a human, discernable in the outline. There was variation in the volume of displacement of the bag. Some were low and flat, indicating slender bodies within, and others showed much more vertical displacement, indicating substantially more volume, usually midway down the length of the bag. This was one of my first real lessons in medical diversity. Of course, I knew that there was great variation in humans and their personal characteristics, but I had never before been responsible for actually recognizing and characterizing those differences and similarities for myself. I would soon be responsible for recognizing tendons and muscles despite their variations in size or sometimes location. This day, however, was in preparation for all of that.

Each anatomy station consisted of a shiny stainless-steel gurney with a body bag atop it. A narrow mobile stainless-steel table spanned the upper thorax and could be adjusted along the gurney by sliding it to expose various parts of the body. Four hard-backed stools, two on each side, completed the teaching setup. We had been given our dissection partners and station assignments in our registration packet. I found my workplace and set down my backpack. I sat in one of the stools and waited as the other students filed in and found their places in a similar fashion. There was a lot of excited chatter, and some of the students were visibly reacting to the laboratory environment. I could tell that this was the first experience with a deceased human for most of the students in the class. At best, some had participated in a course in gross anatomy during their undergraduate studies. I was still dressed in my street clothes, and my white lab coat was still packed in my backpack.

The professors of the class were not present yet. They were having a last-minute meeting, and I had the mental image of this being some sort of a pep talk, standing in a circle and giving a Walmart-style class cheer or chant before jumping into their first day of teaching green first-year students everything they will need to know about the structure of the human body. I noticed a small group of individuals who were already wearing their white lab coats and latex gloves. They were standing in a small circle, discussing something. Shortly, the group broke up, and each went off to a different part of the lab room. The one heading toward my table had a name tag. He got close enough for me to read his identity, and I learned that he was a third-year surgery resident who would be serving as one of the teaching assistants for the course. He approached my table and began to make small talk. His questions were directed at finding out how we were doing in the room full of dead bodies. I told him that it didn't bother me, at all.

We discussed some of my previous experiences, and he ended up asking me if I had ever seen x-rays before. Of course, I had and admitted as much to him. I shouldn't have. He invited me to come and look at some x-rays with him while we all waited for the arrival of the professors. I walked over to the x-ray view box with him, and he reached into a pile of x-rays and pulled out a pair of films. He mounted the two films on the view boxes and turned on the light.

"What do you see?" he asked.

"I don't know" was my response. This was my first day of what would be a tremendous exchange of information and an enormous learning experience, but this was my first day, and my instructor was a surgery resident. What I didn't know was that I was fair game, from the first moment of the first day.

"Well, what do you see?" was the next query.

"An x-ray" came my timid response.

"What part of the body?" followed the next baiting prod.

"It's a chest," I said.

"Male or female?" continued the resident.

"Female" was my determined reply.

"How do you know?" baited the resident. I pointed to the mid-upper part of the film, at the breast's shadows, and tapped the film, too shy to mention the anatomic name of the rounded densities visible on the film.

"You are correct" was the response, "and—she has Emerson-Goodwin's syndrome," he said.

At this moment, my ego rose immensely. Here I was, my first day of med school, and I was already getting one-on-one training by a surgery-resident mentor, and I was going to learn something about one of the myriad of diseases and syndromes that could afflict the human body. Of course, I had never heard of Dr. Emerson or Dr. Goodwin, but the thought flashed through my mind that they must have been great physicians, likely British, based on their names. At some point in their careers, they discovered enough clues about some condition of the body that they were able to classify the condition and publish it, achieving immortality by having their names irrevocably associated with their own syndrome. Was it a fatal condition? What was its cause? I was eager to learn more about this unknown condition. My first real education about a disease. I quickly scanned the x-ray films from top to bottom. I saw the shapes of the lungs and the heart's shadow. I saw the ribs and the diaphragm. I had never really studied any x-rays before, but I was ready to learn. I had not yet learned how to read chest x-rays in an organized fashion. I wasn't clued in to Kerley B lines, an indication of the presence of fluid in and around the lung tissues. Nor was I able to detect differences in the sternoclavicular joints that indicate rotation artifact from the placement of the patient at the time the films were taken. I just saw black, white, and various shades of gray, which gave me the vague idea that this was a chest. But I was willing to learn, so I bit the hook.

"What is Emerson-Goodwin's syndrome?" I asked.

"Well," the resident said, smiling, "that's when you and your buddy are looking at a chest x-ray of a well-developed female and you poke your buddy with your elbow and point to the film and say, 'Hey, 'em are some good ones!'"

It was my first, but not my last, exposure to the unusual sense of humor of surgical residents.

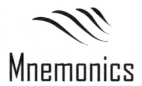

Mnemonics

There was a tremendous amount of information to be learned and retained during medical training. As students, we once calculated the reading time required for our daily assignments, provided that we read at an average pace of "twenty-seven" hours a day. Not only could none of my fellow students ever accomplish such a task, we would never retain that quantity of information. It was apparent to us that we needed help. One of the recognized memory aids taught by psychologists to students to enable them to learn and internally retain information was the use of memory devices called mnemonics. We'd all learned by this method. My earliest mnemonic (pronounced *ni-mo-nik*, silent initial *m*) was in the fourth grade when my teacher enabled me to remember the planets in order with the sentence: "My very extravagant mother just sent us nine parakeets" with the first letter of each word reminding me of a planet.

Now, however, I was learning anatomy and body systems' structure and function. It seemed like mnemonics were everywhere. We were taught some by the residents working in our classes. We made some of them up on our own. Some, like below, were so good that I remember them even to this day.

In the body, there are different types of nerves. There are peripheral nerves that send and receive signals from the spinal cord and other structures within the body. These peripheral nerves follow selected levels and pathways to the extremities and send activating signals to the muscles of that level and receive sensory signals back, to be processed within the spinal cord or forwarded to the higher centers of the brain. Reflexes, such as the type that make your knee jump outward as your kneecap is tapped, are a good example. A sensory nerve to your fingertip is another.

There are, however, a set of twelve special nerves that do not originate from the spinal cord. These twelve nerves originate directly from centers within the brain or upper brainstem and are called cranial nerves. Each of the twelve has associated with it, special functions, some sensory and some motor. They are usually designated by their respective roman numerals and have anatomic names as well. They are—in order, from I through XII—the olfactory, optic, oculomotor, trochlear, trigeminal, abducens, facial, auditory, glossopharyngeal, vagus, accessory, and hypoglossal nerves. The first nerve, for instance, gives us our sense of smell, exquisitely sensitive in the detection of chemical signals within our nose. The eighth nerve gives us a sense of balance and provides our brains with signals interpreted as sound. These important nerves may be remembered, in order, by the rhyming mnemonic: "On old Olympus's towering top, a Finn and German viewed a hop." There is another, more colorful, as well as more memorable one that I recall as well, but that's for another time. Similar memory jingles exist for the eight bones in the wrist, the eight bones of the hind foot, the tendons surrounding the ankle, and many other similar lists of anatomic structures.

Other mnemonic devices are simpler, even single words. In order to remember the order of important structures within the groin crease of the leg, for example, one simply remembers the nearby structure *navel*. When contemplating the procedure of placing a needle within the large femoral vein of the groin—a procedure often employed within the emergency department when fluids are rapidly needed to be given during a resuscitation—the practitioner will expose the groin, clean the skin, and while firmly gripping the large-bore intravenous needle and seeing the belly button, recall that the structures from outside (lateral) to inside (medial) are nerve, artery, vein, empty space, and lymphatics, with the eye finally resting on the *navel*. By feeling for the pulse and placing the entry point medial to that pulse, one is more certain to end up in the vein.

Some mnemonics are nonsensical but, nonetheless, effective memory joggers. For admission orders during my third-year clerkships and beyond (I still use this when admitting a patient, more than thirty years later), I have always relied on the imaginary person's name: DC Van Disselt. This reminds me of each of the elements of the admission orders that I need to put into the patient's chart for completeness. I must write the diagnosis, condition on admission, vital signs frequency, activity level, nursing orders, diet, measurement of intake and output, if needed, special medications, sleep medications, necessary exams, laboratory orders and any other tests required. I don't think anyone has ever met Mr. or Ms. Van Disselt, but DC has saved me many a phone call to clarify a missed or forgotten order.

Finally, sometimes it is just best to recall an ordered list by attaching it to some other well-known list, like the alphabet. We all know our ABCs. Those in emergency services know that, that also stands for the first-three important considerations in an emergency situation: airway, breathing, and circulation. Some EMS instructors continue through DEFG, as well. Most first responders and paramedics are familiar with OPQRST for remembering the essential elements of evaluating a patient's pain as "onset, provokes palliates, quality, radiation, severity and timing." Having never learned the OPQRST mnemonic, I made my own, using LORFCAAT to remind me of "location, onset, radiation, frequency, character, accentuations, alleviations, and timing." Either way, sometimes, in an emergency, it was hard enough to recall the mnemonic to trigger the memory of the actual list to be remembered.

Not all memory devices need to be letters or words. Visual reminders work just as well. Over the years of teaching EMS classes of various levels, I wanted a method to help first responders and paramedics to remember what to do in an emergency situation. Without such a memory jogger, the responder is apt to freeze up at the scene and fail to initiate lifesaving action. Such a person who is present at a scene but fails to take any action has a specific name: *bystander*. In order for my students to keep from simply becoming bystanders at an emergency response, I came up with what I call the Davis Left-Hand Rule of response. I teach my students that, when they arrive at the scene, they have a list of all their important functions right with them, there on their left hands.

If you hold your left hand out, fingers bent in a fist, and the thumb extended, hitchhiking-style, that represents the first step of response to an emergency. Just as the artist uses his extended thumb to *size up* a scene prior to painting it, EMS responders should size up the emergency scene before them prior to taking any action. They should verify that the scene is safe and that they will be safe, as they move in to assist the victims. No downed wires, spilling fuel, chemical contaminants, dangerous traffic, fast-moving water, or other perils should exist that would turn them into another victim. They should, during this brief time, also evaluate how many victims are present and who needs help first.

Next, the index finger is extended, indicating step 2. The index finger is used by most of us to dial the phone. It represents calling for 911 or for other appropriate help. A rule of medicine is "never carry a coffin by yourself," meaning that help or consultation is almost always better than being alone. During my evaluation exams of EMS students, when this step is forgotten, I will, at the end of an evaluation exercise, tell the student to "have a seat while we wait for the ambulance that you never called." Getting an ambulance response early on ensures that you won't be left alone long with a patient who is deteriorating.

I teach my students that the next finger, the middle finger, is the "bad" finger and that bad things can happen to emergency responders who do not protect themselves with personal protective equipment (PPE), such as gloves, gowns, and masks, where appropriate. So at this stage, they know to put on their gloves, at a minimum, and to contain the patient's body fluids to avoid contamination of themselves or others.

The ring finger is next. This response step requires a little anatomic knowledge and association. During anatomy classes, students are taught that within the tube that carries air from the mouth to the lungs, the trachea, there exist cartilage rings that serve to hold the hollow airway tube in an open position. I teach them to associate the word *ring* from the ring finger with the cartilage tracheal rings in order to prompt them that the airway is next up for consideration. Here, they employ other mnemonics, such as ABC and "look, listen, and feel" to help them recall the appropriate actions for securing an adequate airway and ventilation.

Finally, the fifth or "little" finger is extended. During the rapid assessment of an injured person, the upward facing part of the body is readily visible. The examiner can see any blood, traumatic injuries, obvious broken bones, and such. What remains hidden from view is the downward-facing backside. Students are taught, as a part of this step, a *secondary survey*, which is to sweep their hands along the sides of the patient from head to toe, looking for tenderness, deformity, or blood. And if, upon finishing their *blood sweep*, their (gloved, of course) hands show any blood, it is usually found on the lowermost and smallest finger. This *pink on the pinkie* is a sign of hidden injuries to the posterior part of the victim and is prompted by the extended fifth finger.

Use of the Davis Left-Hand Rule will aid an emergency responder in remembering all the essential steps of an emergency response, in an order that will help keep them safe, yet ensure rapid and organized attention to the victim's injuries.

Santa Claus Suit

At the end of the first semester of my first year of medical school, I was unaware as to how quickly the end was approaching. It seemed like the semester had flown by, with experiences piling on other experiences. I had weathered the midterm exams and was in good standing in all my courses. I was also occupied with my work as a teaching assistant in microscopic anatomy. My cadaver had taught me a lot during the five months that passed, and I'd learned many important things about medical school, as well as medicine. Nearing the end of the semester, I developed some confidence in my ability to survive the course of study and to actually thrive within the rigors of the process of becoming a physician. I learned to manage my time and to come to class prepared. I learned to use my evenings and weekends for proper study and review. I even found some time to continue my role as a husband and father. I thought my attitude was even a positive one. One of my classmates, however, must be given the recognition for having the most positive and chipper attitude of all. Near the end of the semester, every student that I knew of was beginning to worry about the upcoming final exam in gross anatomy. We had all diligently attended our lectures each morning. We worked our way through a shelf full of texts of programmed learning of the anatomic structures of the body. We spent most afternoons in the laboratory, working as paired members of a team performing the careful dissection of the human body before us. My partner and I would take turns, one of us reading from the manual and consulting the human anatomy atlas while the other carefully cut away the connective tissue and freed up the anatomic structure that represented our present and immediate concern. We covered the upper and lower extremities and were in the process of completing the abdomen and thorax. We discovered many interesting and unique features of our marvelous "instructor," Nina. I heard many times during the first semester of med school that you never forget three people from your medical training. You never forget the name of your cadaver, the name of the first baby you deliver, and the name of the first person you see die. Nina was in her late sixties and had died in a motor vehicle crash (MVC), at a snowy railroad crossing in northern Iowa. As a last act of compassionate generosity, either she or her family had made a donation of her remains to the anatomic gift program at the University of Iowa. I was one of four direct beneficiaries of that thoughtful gift, as was every patient that I have subsequently provided care for, throughout my career as a physician.

In the process of dissection, we found that Nina had suffered severe chest trauma during the MVC that day. She had multiple fractures on her ribs, resulting in a flail chest. She had one of her lung cavities filled with blood, with the lung collapsed down against the mediastinum. She had contusions on both lungs and a large contusion on her liver. Additionally, we incidentally found benign fibrous tumors on her female organs. She had early atherosclerosis within her coronary arteries and within the lining of her aorta.

With all this learning during that first semester, I was apprehensive about the final exam for the semester, which would be comprehensive, covering any and all material that had been presented during the semester. The final exam would consist of one hundred tables, each containing a cadaver with two labeled items for identification on the test. We would begin the exam at a particular location, all students simultaneously taking their places at their respective dissections, two to a table. We would have a set amount of time, thirty seconds, to identify both structures tagged or otherwise marked at that location and write the answers on our answer sheet, at which time a bell would ring, signaling our transit to the next station of two unknowns. We would proceed around the room, with a visit scheduled at each of the one hundred tables, eventually returning back to our starting point. The two hundred points from this exam contributed significantly toward our final mark for the course.

At the appointed time of the exam, I crammed as much material into my head as I possibly could. I spent most of the prior two weeks reviewing structures, relationships of neighboring landmarks, and even functions of the important anatomy. Despite the preparation, I felt less than ready, mostly due to the sheer volume of the materials covered. I was certain that I looked like the poster child for text anxiety.

I hadn't even given thought to what I would do after final exams were completed. We would finish up just a few days before Christmas, and I'd had no thoughts whatsoever of the impending holidays, having been completely absorbed in the preparations for finals. One of my classmates, however, gave the impression of being completely nonplussed by it all. She showed up to the final exam in fine fashion, wearing a complete Santa Clause outfit, including the beard and hat. I don't know if that outfit aided her in her preparations for or completion of her exam, but her Christmas spirit certainly helped me to relax. She garnered many positive comments about her outfit, including a lot of attention from the exam proctors, one of whom presented to the exam wearing a white T-shirt imprinted with the complete cardiovascular system. He would walk around the exam room, approaching students with his lab coat held open to display the T-shirt logo, saying, "Need any help?" Who would have thought that medical students, so dedicated to learning, would be so fashion-conscious?

Zumbach Suit Story

There are many successful methods of teaching at a medical school, and much is made of the teaching methods of various instructors. Some students, called kinesthetic learners, learn best by physically experiencing the new information. Other students are better at listening to new information and are known as audio learners. Some students are visual learners, doing better at gaining new information if that information is presented in visual form, or in some other form, accompanied by diagrams and illustrations. I tend to float somewhere amid all three. If information is presented to me in audio format, I do best if I can form a mental image of what is being discussed. However, I do similarly well, with direct kinesthetic experience, once I have seen what I am learning or have it explained verbally. One learning experience, however, was pure metaphor. A story, most certainly fictional, that was related to every student in my class, somewhere during my second year of medical school: the Zumbach Suit story.

It seems, according to the story, that a certain businessman had become increasingly successful in his career. As he marked the milestones of his life, he became more and more wealthy, eventually reaching the point where he could afford one of his most hoped-for rewards—a new suit. In his city, there was a tailor who was among one of the most accomplished in his field. His suits were of the finest material and workmanship and were much sought after. The businessman decided the time had come for a new suit, and he had decided that it must be a Zumbach suit.

He made an appointment for the suit measurements and appeared at the appropriate time on the appropriate date. Despite the businessman's excitement, he waited patiently for Mr. Zumbach to show him all the fine fabrics that were stocked for suits. Carefully selecting the material, Mr. Zumbach proceeded to stand the businessman on a wooden crate and moved methodically about him, taking precise measurements of the businessman's neck, shoulders, arms, chest, waist, and leg length, which were recorded on a clipboard, with a pencil retrieved from above Mr. Zumbach's right ear. Following the measurements, the businessman returned to his home and business duties, awaiting word that his suit was ready. Finally, the day came. The long-awaited suit was completed. The businessman returned to the tailors' for the fitting. The suit looked splendid! The lines were clean and crisp. The material was perfectly matched, and the seams were nearly invisible. As the businessman tried on the suit, it felt wonderful. Wearing the suit, he moved to the mirror to inspect the results. The cuffed legs were exactly the right fit, falling just at his heels. The waist was form-fitting, not too tight and not too loose. The jacket was just right around the collar, fitting smoothly down across the shoulders and back. He smartly snapped the sleeves down, first the left and then the right. It was then that he noticed it. The right coat sleeve was two inches too short, falling far back from the shirt sleeve edge, exposing fully two inches of shirt cuff.

This wouldn't do. After spending so much on this article of clothing, the businessman expected nothing less than complete perfection. And Mr. Zumbach, renowned for his suits, wanted nothing less than complete customer satisfaction. Zumbach studied the problem for several moments, then approached the businessman. Placing his hand squarely in the middle of the businessman's right shoulder, he pushed the shoulder forward, forcing the shoulder forward, with a slight twist to his spine and the right arm hanging straight down. This maneuver caused the coat sleeve to slip downward, covering over the exposed shirt cuff.

"Success," said Zumbach.

"Except," said the businessman, "now my coat doesn't fit over my back and shoulders."

Zumbach again studied the man and placed his hand in the middle of the businessman's lower back and bent him forward, releasing the tight collar and shoulders.

"Success again," said Zumbach.

"Wait," said the businessman, "now my pants are touching the floor. My pant legs are too long."

"Well," said Zumbach, "just bend your knees."

The bending of the knees resulted in taking up the slack in the legs, letting the pants cuffs fall at the perfect level. "There," said Zumbach, "a perfect fit." As Zumbach proceeded to shower the businessman with positive comments and accolades regarding the appearance of the once ill-fitting suit. The businessman had to agree that the lengths were all correct but were only that way due to the exotic posture that he was required to maintain. He shuffled out the door and moved awkwardly down the street, knees bent, forward at the waist, slumped forward and toward the right, with his right arm hanging down.

After just a few minutes of walking in this manner, he was approached by a person walking the opposite direction. The newcomer pointed at the businessman and said excitedly, "That suit—it's a Zumbach suit, isn't it?"

The businessman was actually quite pleased that his new suit had garnered such attention in such a short time. "Yes, it is a Zumbach suit," followed by a pause and then, "How did you ever know?"

The bystander immediately responded, "Because Zumbach is the only tailor in the world who could fit a person with your disabilities!"

This story made quite an impression on me and was recalled numerous times over the subsequent two years as I experienced the care delivery of a tertiary teaching facility.

Introduction to Clinical Medicine (ICM)

Second semester of my sophomore year was filled by a course called Introduction to Clinical Medicine, or ICM. This was a comprehensive class that essentially took the medical student through the process of the practice of clinical medicine on a practical basis. This was recognized as the end of the basic sciences, and finally, we were able to learn how to examine patients, talk with patients, take their history, and gather information that would result in the making of a diagnosis and development of a treatment plan. Of course, this was not the first time I'd ever seen a patient because we had had three introductory classes and all of us had experiences during anatomy and physiology with learning about the structure and function of our fellow classmates' bodies. There was even a section on physical examination of the opposite sex that was a coeducational experience with male students examining some of the females in the class and the female students examining some of the males in the class. I personally didn't participate in this, but I know many classmates who found it to be a rewarding experience. During the early part of the semester, each student at the University of Iowa received several gifts that were provided by the Eli Lilly company, including a black leather examination bag, tuning fork, and reflex hammer. This was also the opportunity to purchase an ophthalmoscope of our choosing, which was purchased at a reduced rate for Medical Student Association members. My job was to learn to use these tools in a manner that would be comfortable for the patient as well as provide me the best information toward making a diagnosis.

It was during this ICM class that I first learned the techniques of palpation, percussion, strength testing, and general physical examination. The textbook was a pocket-size handbook written by one of the faculty members and his son that was called *DeGowin and DeGowin's Diagnostic Examination*. This became the bible for physical examination and served as a go-to reference for many, many years. Using my new equipment as well as the pocket reference book, I carefully memorized the steps of examination and then in turn examined my friends, my family members, including my children and wife, and anybody else who would allow me to approach them for examination purposes. I used to look into my wife's eyes with my new ophthalmoscope so much that she would have white afterimages in her visual fields, and never once did she complain. I learned how to use the tuning fork to check hearing and the reflex hammer, of course, to check reflexes and found that I could elicit knee-jerk reflexes quite easily on my wife's lower extremities even without the hammer. All these experiences were valuable in preparation for finally seeing my first patient.

These ICM experiences were supplemented by practice sessions with my classmates, and when it came to more personalized areas, the university even enlisted the help of paid volunteer patients who served as examination subjects for private areas of the body, both male and female. I recall being very apprehensive before each of these experiences because they were after all graded and oftentimes resulted in immediate feedback of success or failure.

During this period, my experience broadened, and I became aware of how my own body responded to examination process. For example, I learned that I could hear my own heartbeat with my stethoscope firmly planted in my ears, which created a distraction when it came to cardiology examinations. I also learned that I had fairly large hands, which, in the future, would be great for catching delivered babies, but not so great for conducting pelvic examinations. In all, I survived this rite of passage with good marks, great experience, and a good, solid preparation to enter the area of clinical medicine.

What Is a Chief Complaint?

One of the terms that is used quite frequently in medicine gener-ally and throughout this book is the term *chief complaint*, and you might be asking yourself, "What is a chief complaint?" The term, as it is taught to every new medical student, means simply "what is the reason for the patient's visit or question?" and is typically identified by the first few words uttered by the patient upon arrival of the visit. In various times in my career, I'd been taught to literally write down word for word what the patient says as the reason for their visit as the chief complaint. In other circumstances, I had to surmise the pur-pose of the visit, particularly if the patient is nonverbal. Sometimes the chief complaint is surmised from comments by others attending the visit.

The chief complaint offers the opportunity to focus the exam and evaluation in a way that just answers a single question or results in a general health checkup that may cover a variety of problems, which are currently noticed or unnoticed. Sometimes the chief com-plaint is awkward. Sometimes it is funny; sometimes it is very sad. However, it directs what happens next and, to an astute examiner, leads to an expedient outcome. Failure to obtain or react appropri-ately to the chief complaint may result in an adverse outcome, the patient's question not being answered sufficiently or lead to misinter-pretation of the patient's intention.

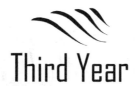

Third Year

Following the two years of basic science education, which consists of studying from books and very little, if any patient contact, the third-year medical student enters the world of clinical rotations. This places the third-year clerk in the situation of actually interviewing patients, collecting and recording histories and physical examinations, and participating in medical decision-making. The rotations last four to six weeks, with some subspecialties lasting just two weeks. My very first rotation began in July of my third year, the same time as new interns arrive at hospitals. Thus, the patient who enters a teaching hospital during the early days of June will be faced with a medical staff that is fresh, young, and inexperienced. My very first rotation gave me the assignment of psychiatry at Veteran's Administration Hospital.

First Day with VA Patient

The very first day of clinical work started off with an orientation meeting for all third-year students. We met in a large auditorium, where we reviewed the expectations of the rotations, an introduction to the daily schedules, and to remind us of the presence of *real patients* in our lives from this point forward. The Veteran's Administration Hospital was just a couple hundred yards from the college of medicine, and I walked briskly to the site of my first clinical experience. I had worked toward this goal for six years of higher education. I wore my newly issued white coat and carried my recently gifted black physician's bag. I had a shirt and tie on and was prepared to immerse myself in the total experience of being a real health-care provider. I arrived on the psych ward, the ninth floor of the hospital, just after ten. The new residents and interns had been there since seven that morning and were already busily beginning their new rotations. I found the offices within the ward by asking for directions twice along the way. In the office, I found my first intern, whom I'll call Dr. M. The intern Dr. M. was just a couple of years my senior and looked it. He also had a shirt and tie and sat behind the desk, a world away from me in terms of experience and power. "Great," he said, as we finished the introductions. "Your first patient is waiting in the exam area," he continued, pointing to a room with a closed door.

With great trepidation, I gathered up my things and headed for the door. This was the moment, at last. I'd wanted to be a physician for a long time. I'd sweated through all of that premed competitiveness and through the admissions process. I'd made it through the first two years of labs and didactics. Now I was reaching for the door handle for my very first real patient.

Well, of course, I'd had practice patients during my Introduction to Clinical Medicine (ICM) course the prior semester, but this was my very first actual patient—a psychiatric patient. Would it be depression? Suicide? Psychosis? Dependency? I realized that it could be any number of things, or even something that I hadn't learned about yet. What then? How would I know what questions to ask? Well, the intern would help me, I'm sure. The basic history and physical would be the same regardless of the complaint. I opened the door. There, in a T-shirt and gray sweatpants sat my patient. A young black man of large stature sat there on the chair, staring at the door as I entered. He certainly wasn't smiling. Was that a glare? I wasn't sure. I sat down in the only other chair in the room after sliding it across the room to a position that was facing him.

"Hello, I'm Jim Davis, a third-year medical student. I'd like to interview you for your admission to the hospital today." He gave no discernable response, either verbal or nonverbal, and yes, that was a glare. "What brings you to the Veteran's Hospital today?" I asked, starting with the simple open-ended question that I'd been taught and had practiced over and over.

"They sent me here from St. Louis" was his short and to-the-point reply. Not much information, but it was a start.

"The St. Louis VA sent you here?" I asked.

Yes was the terse reply. I wasn't learning much from him very quickly. I didn't know how much time I had for the interview, but I suspected that it wasn't all day.

"Why did the St. Louis VA send you here?" I asked. In my mind, I imagined that the doctors at the St. Louis hospital had simply run across an illness that they couldn't manage and had, in their wisdom, recognized the superiority of the doctors and hospital system where I was training and referred their difficult problem to the more competent hospital for evaluation, diagnosis, and treatment. Certainly, the VA hospital in St. Louis could recognize quality, as could everyone else in the Midwest.

"Well," he began, "they kicked me out of the hospital in St. Louis because I beat up one of their doctors."

My jaw must have dropped because I noticed his smile at me as he knew that he had made an impression on me.

"What did you do?" I asked, hoping that I had misunderstood him.

"I hit him with a pool cue," he said, leaning forward toward me. He was larger than me, and although I was in pretty good shape from some not-too-long ago participation in intercollegiate football, I had no desire to mix it up with him on a hospital ward. I decided to change the subject quickly, back to the information that I needed to finish my job.

"What illness brought you to the hospital in St. Louis in the first place?" I queried.

"I have bipolar," replied the patient, finally giving me some information that I could use. Through the subsequent history taking, I learned all about his previous hospitalizations, medicines, allergies, family history, social history, and review of systems. I learned, for example, that he served in the Air Force for a short time and spent some time in Vietnam. I also learned that he had had gonorrhea, but that it had been treated while he was in the military. I finished my detailed history and began my physical exam. Again, this was the first time I'd done this for real. I drew upon all my (limited) prior experience. I took his vital signs, not knowing that the nurse had already done the same thing. I listened carefully to his lungs, his heart, and his abdomen. I peered curiously into his ears, nose, and throat. I palpated and percussed his abdomen and flank. While he was lying down, I carefully checked his hips, knees, and ankles. Other than some superficial scars, I saw nothing out of the ordinary.

As he lay in the supine position, I looked around the room and saw the rubber gloves and donned them prior to examining his genitalia. I then reached for the lubricating gel and the blood detection card (guaiac card) that is used to screen for rectal cancer. He was rather young to be a cancer candidate, but I'd been warned that a complete physical was required on every patient and that it was not acceptable to cut corners by skipping the rectal exam, particularly at the Veteran's Administration Hospital. My training had been good, and I had no intention on cutting corners.

"I need to check your prostate," I said, in my best composed voice. "I'll need you to drop your shorts and turn a little onto your side."

He immediately sat bolt upright, with such speed that I leaped back a little, out of surprise.

"No way!" he said, his voice raised and agitated. "No way you're gonna put your finger in my butt," he repeated. "That's what that doctor in St. Louis tried to do 'afore I hit 'em with the pool cue—and I'll do the same to you if you try to do that thing to me."

He had by now jumped down to the floor and stood there, in just his boxer shorts, agitated and beginning to pace back and forth. He continued a tirade against the physician at the St. Louis hospital who had tried to "assault" him so perversely. I wasn't certain what to do. I reassured him that I would be right back and reached around for the doorknob and my exit from the threat within the room. I quickly walked through the door, closing it behind me. My heart pounded in my chest, and my fear gave me a lump in my throat. My very first patient had already threatened me with physical harm. I must have looked a little pale and anxious when I found the intern and began my breathless recital of my experience. When I got to the part about the threats, he simply smiled at me.

"I'll tell you what you do," Dr. M. began very calmly. "You take your necktie off and put your stethoscope away, so he can't choke you with them." I didn't like where this was going. "And you go back in there and finish your exam," he finished. Obviously, he didn't believe me. He was sending me back into my doom.

"Okay" came my brief and timid reply. After all, I was just a brand-new third-year student. What did I know? Certainly, my intern had all the answers. I don't remember how I convinced myself to go back into that room. I do remember truly feeling that I might be in danger by doing so. I went back in, without my necktie and without my stethoscope. I told Dr. M. to listen at the door and be ready to rescue me, if I needed it. As I reentered the room, I saw that my patient now sat, still in his boxers, back on the chair.

"You're not gonna do that check on me, are you?" was his first question. Or maybe it was not a question; maybe it was an order. I could only tell the truth.

"I have to," I said. "The intern wants me to check you," I continued, trying to think my way out of this situation. I could see that, although he had calmed down while I was out of the room, he would heat up again very quickly.

"Why? Why do you have to do that check?" he asked, standing up next to the exam table to meet me face-to-face.

"Because you had gonorrhea," I said, thinking of the only thing that came to mind. "And gonorrhea can hide out in the prostate and come back to infect you again if it is not treated properly."

He immediately spun around, faced the exam table, bared his bottom toward me, leaned over, and placed his hands on the table, saying, "Gonorrhea? Man, that's bad crap! Anything, doc, you can do anything to me, jus' don't make me have gonorrhea again."

I was so surprised at his action that I stood there for a moment, wondering what to do. Before he changed his mind, I quickly placed gel on my gloved finger and completed the exam. I even got a small quantity of stool for analysis for unseen blood. Finished, I handed him a tissue and quietly told him that was the end of the exam. He began to change as I left the room, astonished at my success.

"How'd it go?" came the question from Dr. M. as I went to pick up my necktie and stethoscope.

"Oh, it all came out all right once he knew who was in charge," I said, holding back a smile.

First Day, Code Blue

I really don't remember much else about my time on the ward that first day. I remember that I finished up around 5:00 p.m. and headed back to the medical school. The medical school was literally just across the street from the VAH, but the adjacent parking lots made the walk a lot longer. The college of medicine administrative offices flanked the eastern side of the large teaching hospital and shared a common parking lot with the emergency department ambulance entrance. Over the previous months of medical school, I had often exited the administrative offices, the location of all the med student's mailboxes, only to see an ambulance parked in front of the ED entrance. I had never seen an actual ambulance turn into the lot, nor had I ever seen ambulance personnel in the parking lot, just the parked vehicle. Presumably, the intermittent presence of the vehicle meant that some lifesaving event was occurring within the walls of the hospital, with lives hanging in the balance and medical personnel anxiously engaged in salvaging some human specimen therein. I had grown up with the television show *Rescue 911* with paramedics Johnny Gage and Roy Desoto rushing around Southern California accident scenes and speeding off to Rampart General Hospital with the latest of the sick and afflicted called for in their weekly script. I knew that, on the show, at least, Dr. Brackett and Nurse McCall had everything well in hand and, rarely, if ever, lost a patient. Surely that's what emergency medicine was all about. My turn to learn the truth would come much later in the year, the last of my third-year rotations, in fact, when I would join the Surgery Department, in June of the next year, for a six-week stint to include covering the ED. So any ED experience was a long way off, for me, or so I thought. As I turned from the sidewalk into the parking lot and headed for the double doors that led to the college of medicine medical student mail room, I was carrying my black doctor's bag, with all my new examination and diagnostic equipment, my mind on the events of the day, and I surmised that I'd have a lot to tell my family about my first day of my clerkships.

My daydream was interrupted by a car that turned from the street into the parking lot of the hospital ED, narrowly missing me as it sped past. It pulled up to the automatic doors of the ED and screeched to a stop outside; the driver repeatedly honking his horn. As I approached the car casually, from behind and close to the passenger side, the driver leaped out and said, "Yes, help him. He's a cardiac patient!" Now recall that I had exactly one day's experience with real patients, and I had not yet had internal medicine, where we students would be taught the techniques of advanced cardiac life support. I had been taught basic CPR, however, and as I quickened my steps toward the passenger door, I saw for the first time that the front seat contained an elderly gentleman, slumped toward the car door, with his face awkwardly resting against the car window. His eyes were closed, and he looked ashen gray. The driver ran around the back of the car, and as he headed toward the double automatic-open doors, he again shouted. "Help him! He's a cardiac patient." I dropped my bag and white coat onto the pavement and grasped the door handle.

"Go in and get help," I said. "I'll get him out of the car." As the driver burst through the doors, I opened the passenger door, and the patient slowly leaned further out of the door toward the pavement. I caught his shoulders, keeping him from sprawling onto the ground, and used gravity to aid me in getting him out of the car. He wasn't breathing, and he had no muscle tone whatsoever. He was just floppy and slid out of the car onto the pavement. I checked for a pulse and felt none. The BLS training that I'd received had taught me to check for breathing and then for pulses. He had neither. I knew that the next step was to begin mouth-to-mouth breathing. This was in the era before AIDS, personal protective equipment and body substance isolation and M-T-M was the recommended airway technique. I'd learned it but had never practiced it. I had seen it done on *Rescue 911*, however, and it was almost always successful, enabling Johnny and Roy to wheel through the doors of Rampart General with a salvageable patient. This was the real thing. Admittedly without much thought or concern, I took a deep breath, tilted this man's mouth open, placed my mouth over the mouth of a complete stranger, pinched his nose, and blew in. There was a short period of resistance, followed by a slow flow of air from my lungs into his. His chest rose up, and I broke my contact with his mouth. A rush of air followed, as my breath escaped from his lungs. I was just preparing to give my second breath when I heard a commotion behind me. The double doors burst open, and several people, all dressed in the white uniforms of hospital staff and guiding a wheeled table, ran quickly toward me. I turned and looked toward them, seeing the urgency in their faces as they came to a stop next to me. Two young men grasped the old man's shirt by the shoulders, and a third grabbed his feet, expertly lifting him and sweeping him onto the gurney in a fluid motion. They ran the several steps back to the double doors and disappeared inside. I stood there next to the car, watching as the driver came out of the ED doorway and walked toward the car.

"I guess I'd better move this," he said, rather sadly, moving toward the driver's door. The car was still running; I noticed. I couldn't understand his dejected attitude. Obviously, he didn't know of the magnificent abilities of the emergency personnel within those walls. On TV, they rarely lost a patient. Certainly, real life must be no different. Besides, this was a fantastic teaching hospital where godlike specialists performed feats of heroic medical magic on a daily basis.

As I walked across the parking lot toward the medical school entrance, I reviewed the events that had just transpired once again in my mind. I felt some dissatisfaction at my clumsiness in providing CPR, wishing that there were more that I could have done. I felt admiration for the well-trained team that had intervened, literally snatching the patient from me, whisking him into the mysterious confines of the hospital ED. I felt that I could probably never know enough medicine to be a contributing part of a team like that. Besides, I had no interest in emergency medicine.

He's Not a Real Doctor

Psychiatric units are great sources for stories about medicine and patients. I think it is the natural tendency for those of us who are of "normal" thought to find humor and entertainment in the lives of those who live near or over the edge. Perhaps we see just how close we are to being over the imaginary line into the realm of pathologic thought, or perhaps we are simply intrigued by how someone else could look at the world that we find strange, bizarre, or frightening, and see it as normal and acceptable. Anyway, spending just a short time on a behavioral unit (psych ward) can be very, very educational, both from the viewpoint of observing and learning the vast array of illness that can befall our minds, but also by gaining insight as to what constitutes "normal" and how to recognize abnormalities of thought. Some of the humor of these stories comes because of the surprising level of insight and thought that is evident within patients who are supposedly not functioning at a very high level.

My first clerkship as a third-year student came on the behavioral unit of a veteran's hospital. Sadly, some of these patients, by far comprised of men at that time, were being hospitalized for posttraumatic illness, depression, and the effects of alcohol or drug addiction from the era of the Vietnam War and the Korean War. The old-timers were often emphysematous and stroke or renal patients from World War II. While attending to the needs of the ward one day, I looked up from the chart that I was updating when a commotion began in the center of the large open main room of the unit. It was a room that contained tables and chairs, a television, a pool table, and various other recreational items. The patients generally either sat at the tables playing cards or board games or conversing or milled about in a slow shuffle that took them essentially nowhere quickly, sometimes stopping by the windows to look out at the weather. The ward was on the ninth floor, so the view was pretty good, unless you actually wanted to see trees and flowers. One could watch the thunderstorms roll in over the Midwestern flatlands, however, and the lightning provided for some spectacular light shows when it stormed. Anyway, the whole place was really like something out of *One Flew Over the Cuckoo's Nest*, complete with a middle-aged registered nurse of mean temperament, who was typecast for Nurse Ratchet.

A group of men had gathered in the center of the room where a single patient lay on the floor in the midst of a grand mal convulsion. I dropped my pen and leaped from my seat, running to the knot of people bent over, looking down at the helpless victim. One of the other patients was bent over, kneeling beside the downed and convulsing man, gown askew, telling the gathered bystanders that he was a doctor and that they should all "stand back and give me some room." He asked further whether anyone knew CPR. I arrived just at the same time as the intern who, was coming from a different direction, kneeled down beside the "doctor" in the patient gown and quietly told him that I could take over for him now. I quickly assessed the patient's airway and breathing while the intern checked for a pulse. I knew that the patient had a history of seizures and suspected that his medication level had somehow declined to the point that the seizure became possible. Patients were known to hide their medications under personal belongings, to save them for an overdose, to sell to other patients, or simply because they were tired of taking them. The patient's seizure activity slowed and then stopped, with the patient's arms lying flaccidly at his side. His breathing returned to a regular pattern. I carefully wiped the saliva from his lips and opened his mouth cautiously with a wooden tongue depressor, taking care to keep my fingers clear of his teeth in case he suddenly clenched his jaws. The uncontrolled biting could easily result in the loss of a finger. His airway was clear, and his breathing was now normal. His body was resting quietly as a result of his muscles being fatigued from the recent eruption of uncontrolled neurological impulses from his brain, relaxing, exhausted, and nearly incapable of further contractions. I positioned his head to allow for easier flow.

I overheard the displaced "doctor" telling the gathered bystanders, "He's not really a doctor…He's just pretending," pointing to me with a nicotine-stained finger.

I chuckled to myself, hoping that the intern had not overheard. The intern looked up at me with the beginnings of a grin and said, "That guy is exactly right about you. Are you sure he even needs to be in here?"

Ivan

Another patient on that same ward taught me an immensely valuable course in disordered thought. John was a tall, slender young man from a farming background. He also had a profound psychosis, a thought disorder that had caused his parents to bring him to the hospital for a prolonged stay. When I first went in to meet him, he was plainly dressed in a work shirt, blue jeans, white socks, and well-worn lace-up work boots. He sat in a chair, with a huge grin on his face as I introduced myself and sat down for our interview. He spoke plainly, without any pressure or rush to his speech. Just a rural drawl and plain words that made him simple and likeable. The only thing that I noticed immediately was that he turned his head often during his answers and seemed a little uneasy when my questions ventured beyond the simple questions of name, address, phone, and the like. I noted his uneasiness and asked him if he was comfortable in that chair. His reply was that he would be more comfortable in another chair and pointed across the room at a desk chair, pushed into the kneehole of a desk. I thought that it might be softer or adjustable in a way that he found attractive, so I got up and brought the chair with roll, tilt, and swivel functions over to our spot and invited him to trade up. He did so readily and sat there facing me, gently rocking back and forth a little in his new seat. As I asked him some more questions, I became aware that his previously noted head turning now became a movement of his whole body, turning to the left each time he answered a question. He would then turn back to face me after his answer, always with a calm, pleasant look and quiet voice.

I said "John, I've noticed that you turn your chair away from me when you answer my questions. Is there a particular reason for that?"

He smiled and said, "Yes, I have to face the northeast when I answer your questions."

"Why is that?" I queried.

"Because all my power comes from the northeast, and I need that power to think of the answers to your questions" came the surprising reply.

Over the next several minutes of questioning, the depth of John's thought disorder became evident to me. He was having auditory and visual hallucinations, hearing voices and seeing things that no one else could hear or see. He had never become violent but had simply ceased to function, stopping frequently to listen to what the voices were telling him, staring off at some unseen object that held his fascination for a few moments. He had suffered some accidents on the farm because of his inattention, and his parents had begun to consider him a threat of self-harm, albeit accidental, because of his frequent close calls with farm machinery while listening and seeing the unseen and unheard. John spent several weeks on the inpatient unit while his medications were adjusted and new medicines tried by the attending psychiatrists.

One day, while out on a walk with a recreation therapist, John discovered "gold" and brought back a cowboy hat full of what appeared to me to be common driveway gravel. But in each piece, John saw and could point to a thin vein of gold, "plain as day." He carefully stored his "gold" in his dresser drawer, lest one of his friends on the ward make off with his treasure. Oh, and the cowboy hat—it was bright red and had an adjustable tie that fit under his chin just like the cowboy hats of my childhood. I didn't even know that they made them that big, but he had one. He was very, very proud of it, until another patient happened to mention that it might just be a little too bright red in color and that he should "tone it down a bit." John's response was to carefully apply a camouflage pattern to the brim and center with liquid brown shoe polish. He wore that red and brown hat every day, taking it off only at bedtime. I think he even wore it into the shower. On his medications, he gradually improved and became more conventional in his thought and actions. Even when he no longer felt the necessity to turn toward the northeast to answer questions, he still maintained that that compass direction was his source of power. He actually lived in a community that was geographically located north and east of the hospital, so perhaps he was right.

Psych Rotation, Falling Asleep

As I mentioned, my first rotation as a third-year student was on the psychiatry service. I was assigned to the psychiatric inpatient unit at the VA Hospital, which was located adjacent to the vast university hospital's campus and connected to the university hospital by an underground tunnel system. This allowed the easy transfer of patients, students, and staff between the two hospitals, even during poor weather. All the students, regardless of their assigned location, would meet for a weekly conference with a staff physician. During this conference, students might listen to a presentation by a respected staff member, hear a conference between residents, or make a presentation of one of their own patients to an attending staff physician. In addition to my duties as a student, I was employed by the hospital laboratory system as a provider of laboratory technical services.

My specific responsibility was in the newborn intensive care, where I provided services that included the obtaining and analysis of newborn blood for determining the amount of oxygen and carbon dioxide that it contained (blood gas analysis). More modern techniques allow for this to be determined by an external clip on probe that is applied to the newborn's toe, finger, or earlobe, but at the time, such noninvasive abilities did not yet exist. The usual method was to obtain a blood sample from the heel or finger of a newborn. Because the fingers and toes were very fragile, they were very rarely used, and a poke of the skin of the heel was more commonly the source of the blood specimen.

Newborns are prone to breathing problems as a major source of complications, especially any babies that are born prematurely. Lungs are some of the last organs to reach maturity and do so just before birth. When a birth occurs early, it is often accompanied by immature lungs, which do not exchange oxygen very well. As a result, the baby breathes very quickly, which requires great effort and places a great strain on the baby's heart and brain. Because oxygen, while vital for all living organisms, can be toxic if given in too high of a concentration, the levels of oxygen in premature newborns must be monitored very carefully.

It was my job to help in this monitoring by directly measuring levels of oxygen, carbon dioxide, and the buildup of acid in the blood of preemies. This lab was staffed twenty-four hours a day, and while a student, I covered the lab on the overnight shift, from 11:00 p.m. to 7:00 a.m. For some reason, hospital employees resisted calling this by its more common term: *the graveyard shift.*

It was on the morning following one of these shifts that I was scheduled to attend a weekly meeting with my team of fellow third-year students with the attending psychiatrist. It was my turn to present a patient to the attending. During this presentation, the student would generally review all the patient's pertinent history—his life story up to that point. We would relate the patient's background, the events leading up to the admission, the patient's prior medical and psychiatric history, as well as all the significant events in the patient's family, medical, and psychiatric backgrounds. Following this delivery of information, the attending psychiatrist would then ask the patient further questions to clarify any of the presentation or to correct anything that was not clear at that point. Literally, any topic or question was open for the asking to either the patient under discussion or the student presenter.

I had chosen a particularly interesting patient with the diagnosis of schizophrenia. This gentleman, in his late forties, was severely afflicted and had been so for many years. His delusions and hallucinations were very well ingrained, and he interacted very abnormally with his environment. Most often, he could be found speaking to himself or to invisible others, hearing responses from unseen speakers, and reacting to the commands of those voices who were controlling him. The modern term for this behavior is *responding to internal stimuli.* I believe that he had a whole imaginary world going on inside his head. I recall that I was very, very tired as I made my presentation of this man's history. I had practiced all night, when my lab-tech duties would allow me, and I had most of his history memorized. I was certain that it was a flawless delivery. The attending, the patient, and I were all seated in a small circle, with the other members of my team seated nearby, behind the patient's chair. I remember finishing my presentation of the history and the attending turning to the patient and asking a single question about his home. I was not certain exactly what happened next. However, the next thing that I was aware of was a member of my team touching me on my left shoulder and saying my name. "Jim?"

I then heard the attending say, "Can the patient tie his own shoes?"

Apparently, this was the fourth time the attending had asked me that question. I had fallen asleep, sitting completely upright, with my eyes open, completely unaware of my surroundings. At the third repetition of the attending's question, my classmate had stood, walked over, and placed his hand on my shoulder to awaken me. Fortunately for me, I didn't startle or jump. I simply answered yes, and my classmates later told me that it appeared as though I was just thinking about the question. However, the attending had been questioning the patient for three or four minutes before turning to me with his question. I had likely been dozing the whole time. It was at that moment that I learned that I could sleep nearly anywhere, at nearly any time. If the attending ever noticed my lapse, he never mentioned it. I was careful to watch my schedule thereafter and tried not to allow a shift on a night prior to any serious academic assignment.

Pit Drip

Typically, teaching hospitals look to the labor force of their students in order to maximize the financial benefit to the teaching program. That is, in addition to the tuition paid by the student, there is the expectation, by the institution, that the student will serve as a part of the necessary patient-care workforce. Recently, constraints have been placed upon the number of hours required of the house staff. Schools have long recognized the constraints of the student labor force brought about by their minimal level of training and all the competing demands placed upon their time. This does not always prevent the expectations from being made, nonetheless. One example of this would be the infamous "pit drip" on obstetrics.

Now mothers have been having children for a long, long time. They've been historically successful for the most part, without the presence of an obstetrician, trained obstetrical nurses, and certainly without medical students. Modern medicine tends to intervene during the labor process a little more often, in hopes of decreasing infant mortality and morbidity. This intervention takes on many forms, such as slowing or stopping preterm labor, augmentation of dwindling labor contractions, or even "starting" someone into labor before their natural processes start up. The latter two of these, augmenting or beginning labor means that the attending physician introduces into the woman's body a manmade form of the natural hormone that produces labor (Pitocin or "pit") via an intravenous line placed for that purpose. This hormone, which occurs physiologically in the pituitary, is released in response to the late stages of pregnancy and brings about rhythmic contractions of the muscles of the uterus and, hopefully, expulsion of the baby. When this hormone is introduced in artificially higher quantities, the patient and particularly her womb must be carefully monitored to be certain that the hormone level is adequate to accomplish the onset and maintenance of regular contractions, but not so high a level as to cause unrelenting contractions of the uterus or even tearing of the muscular uterine wall, which would certainly be perilous to the passenger inside.

Modern medicine accomplishes this monitoring with a bit of rather crafty technology. A small plastic box, the tocodynamometer (*toco*, meaning "uterine;" *dyno,* "movement;" *meter*, "measurement") that contains a simple spring-loaded button, is placed upon the mom's tummy. Enough tension is applied with elastic belts that the pressure of the button makes a slight depression in the normal skin of the woman's pregnant abdomen. During a contraction, this skin tightens due to the rigidity that develops in the uterine wall, sitting immediately beneath the skin, and this tight skin pushes out against the button, displacing it and causing it to electronically register the contraction. Because the contraction gradually builds up and then diminishes, this signal takes the shape of a rounded hump in the line of recording ink. Also recorded on the same sheet of paper or electronic record is the heart rate of the soon-to-be-newborn. Analysis of the heartbeat's variation in the context of the contraction enables the baby attendant to assess the amount of stress being experienced by the fetus. That's the new technology. The old technology consisted of placing a hand on the mother's abdomen and feeling for the contraction and placing a special stethoscope (having the appearance of a unicorn horn) on the abdomen and listening carefully for the baby's heartbeat and counting the beats to determine the baby's pulse rate at several times before, during, and after the contraction. The truth is, the teaching institution where I trained as a student was on the cutting edge of the technology and had acquired several of the new machines for use in fetal monitoring. The nurses used them during the day shifts, when students were in class or on rounds. At night, however, the machines were set aside, and each student who was on rotation to labor and delivery was placed in a chair beside the bed of a laboring mother who was receiving the Pitocin hormone, given a clipboard with a blank labor record on it, a pen, and a clock with a sweep hand to time and record each contraction. We were the fetal monitors. Remember that the average first-time labor is sixteen hours, and these mothers were already, by definition, not average. They were receiving the artificial hormone because their labors were prolonged or nonexistent. Thus, the med student needed to sit at the bedside, stay awake, record all the labor contractions accurately, and then stand in for the actual delivery, perhaps many hours later. Because the student was at the patient's bedside and could take vital signs, the nurses were free to do other things. Mostly, they sat in the nurses' station and chatted. It was very boring with nothing to do between the contractions except fight to stay awake. The room was dimmed, so the mom could doze between contractions, so reading or studying was out of the question. I hated pit drips. The main thing that kept my interest was my anticipation of having obstetrics be a part of my future practice.

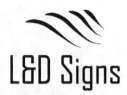

L&D Signs

One of the required rotations during the third year was to spend time on labor and delivery. In addition to developing an interest in having obstetrics be a part of my future practice, I learned a couple of valuable lessons while on the service. The main area of the unit was set up with a long countertop, which was used for medical students to write their postdelivery notes in the chart. These notes were the responsibility of the medical student or resident during the delivery and were meant to contain such information as the progression of labor, the actual delivery time, any complications of the delivery, any instrumentation that had to occur—such as, vacuum extraction, forceps, the position of presentation of the fetus, estimated blood loss, a description of the umbilical cord—such as, knots, number of vessels in the cord, Apgar scores, necessary resuscitation of the infant, and other pertinent facts. This became the definitive record of the birth of that infant and was therefore an official hospital record.

There were a couple of noteworthy signs posted immediately above the writing area at that desk site. One of them was the warning "You can put any child through any pelvis, but try to put them through the third grade." This rather dark humor was directed at trying to avoid any unnecessary or dangerous intervention for the delivering mother. Another additional word of wisdom was presented in a similar sign that said, "Don't just do something, stand there." Medical students during the course of writing their notes were constantly presented with these two bits of wisdom to remind that for thousands of years, young women had been delivering babies successfully without the intervention offered by a third-year medical student. This natural process would oftentimes proceed if simply left alone and unimpeded. During the course of their rotation as well as the first few years of my active practice, I recalled these two pieces of beneficial information on many occasions. The author, although unknown, certainly imparted a lot to my education.

This first experience with labor and delivery taught me a couple of other things in addition to ensuring that I wanted to include the delivery of newborns and their aftercare in the scope of my practice. My first delivery experience was with my own private family physician in the delivery of my third daughter, Amy, at the private hospital across town from the university. My wife went into labor in mid-September, and when we arrived at the hospital, labor was already well-established. As my wife progressed to the later stages of labor, the doctor upon his arrival said, "*Ooh* you're the medical student, do you want to deliver this one?"

Over the next several minutes, I told him that I had not previously delivered any babies. He assured me that he could talk me through it. Therefore, I was already one delivery ahead of most of my classmates. Nonetheless, I soon found that I had much to learn in the area of labor and delivery, progressing through the learning experiences shared in common with my classmates, including monitoring active labor contractions, determining cervical effacement and dilation, stimulation of stalled labor with Pitocin, management of the third stage of labor, routine episiotomy repair, and aftercare of the mother. In a university teaching program, electronic monitors were a fairly new invention, as I had previously mentioned, and were really unnecessary because we had multiple medical students with nothing else to do except to sit by laboring women with their hands on the women's tummies to establish the pattern of labor contractions. What I learned was that labor consisted of a lot of time spent closely watching laboring mothers followed by a rapid crescendo to a near crisis level at the time of delivery followed by, in most cases, extreme joy of new motherhood. There were not many situations that resolve themselves so completely or with such immediate gratification. Almost all the results of labor were positive with the extreme discomfort of delivery resolving itself rapidly, and no one to receive credit but the attending doctors. With this experience also came the study and understanding of the women's estrous cycle, contraception, delivery, and aftercare. I came through my obstetrics first rotation with several additional deliveries and a generalized understanding of the mechanical process of delivery and its potential complications as well as the need for immediate intervention and a healthy respect for the natural delivery process. Knowing what the potential complications of delivery of even a healthy newborn could present, I also developed a healthy respect for the availability of intervention to be immediately available during even apparently uncomplicated deliveries. This later allowed me to adopt the opinion that "home deliveries are for pizzas" and should not generally be entertained by expectant mothers.

One of the third-year rotations that I was required to do was anesthesia. This allowed me to experience the operating room environment on a different level and added to my prior experiences and surgery. I learned that anesthesia had a reputation of being a profession for which the practice of sheer boredom was occasionally punctuated by brief episodes of stark terror.

One memorable event from this phase of my training was the day I learned about the oculocardiac reflex. This is a reflex that is apparently well-known by everyone except third-year medical students. In order to elicit this reflex, a surgeon puts pressure on the side of the globe of the eye causing it to shift position, and this elicits a profound slowing of the heart rate (bradycardia) followed by an immediate drop in blood pressure. I thought I had read all the pertinent information prior to going to the operating room for the first day but still didn't catch on when the surgeon looked at my supervising anesthesiologist with a gleam in his eye and said, "You think we should teach the medical student about the oculocardiac reflex?" And because of a surgical mask, I didn't see his smile. I was listening to the patient's heartbeat through my anesthesia stethoscope and suddenly heard the heartbeat interrupted by long pauses of the produced bradycardia. I knew the antidote for slow heart rate was to administer atropine and was nonetheless reminded of this fact by my mentor when he handed me the vial of atropine and told me the appropriate dose. This readily resolved the crisis and taught me a valuable lesson about bradycardia and eye surgeons.

Urology, Hypothyroid Patient

One thing that the third year of medical school teaches you is how to be very thorough when you interview a patient. This is achieved by a variety of means, including practice interviews with patients who then review your history and exam with the instructors. The result is that the physical exam and history-taking procedures are committed to memory. It is true that later, you will learn which questions are low-yield and which are not. You also learn, somewhere along the way, to do a somewhat directed history, asking questions generally and then going more in depth when some positive responses lead you in that direction. The fact is, during your third year, before any forgetfulness or corner-cutting sets in, you probably are at your peak in doing a complete history and physical. This can sometimes lead you to some unusual outcomes.

While on the urology service, I had a patient that will always remind me of what is possible when a complete H&P is done. Raymond was a resident at one of the state hospitals that provided care for individuals with mental or severe psychological handicaps that prevented them from thriving in the mainstream society. He had never been circumcised as an infant and had, as an adult, suffered through a series of increasingly serious infections of the glans, with the medical name of balanitis. This was not only painful for Raymond but caused a significant increased need for nursing care for the staff of the residential institution. He was therefore sent to the teaching hospital, to the urology department, for an adult circumcision. This would be performed under a general anesthetic the day following his admission. I was given the assignment of doing Raymond's preoperative H and P. Raymond spoke very slowly and had a deep mellow voice that radiated his overall cheerful attitude and friendly demeanor. He was quite a large man and reminded me a great deal of Lenny from *Of Mice and Men*. While he did seem to have a very low intelligence level, he was easy to interview and had a pretty good memory. There was a part of the H and P where the examiner basically reviews all the functioning parts of the body to determine if there was any history of difficulties or malfunctioning in those systems. In fact, it was called a review of systems. I had completed Ray's history up to that point and had begun his review of systems. I knew that Ray worked in the institution's kitchen, as a baker, having obtained that bit of information during my questions about his social history. It came as a surprise to me, then, when I asked a standard question about temperature tolerance, related to the functioning of the thyroid gland. The thyroid gland is an organ that produces thyroid hormone, which helps to regulate the body's metabolism rate. People with overactive thyroid glands are often found to feel warm when the surroundings are in reality normal or cold. Conversely, people with underactive thyroid glands are more likely to be cold in normal environments.

My question to Raymond was Do you ever feel warm when others are normal or cool, or do you ever feel cold when others are normal or warm? Looking back on it, it was a pretty complex question to ask someone whom I've already assessed as being simple-minded, but I had built up some confidence in his ability to understand and answer my questions.

Ray surprised me when he looked at me for a moment, and then in a very slow drawl, said, "Well, I work in a bakery. Oh, I told you that. And I always wear a sweater. Winter or summer, I wear a sweater there in the bakery, right by the ovens. The other guys say I'm silly because I wear a sweater while I'm standing next to the ovens in the summertime. They think I'm crazy because they're sweating and I'm not, and I'm in a sweater."

I thought to myself, *Hmm. I wonder if he could have a thyroid problem.*" I jotted down a note to remind myself to order a thyroid screening test on him when I ordered his pre-op lab work.

Later on, I couldn't find any enlargement of his thyroid gland in the front of his neck, but I noticed that he had thick, coarse hair on his arms and his reflexes seemed a little slow when I tapped on his arms and legs to check them. I had never seen a case of low thyroid function, and I was sure that, given the fact that Raymond was in a residential medical unit and was surrounded by medical staff on a daily basis, his thyroid function had been checked and rechecked numerous times. I even had to ask the intern which test to order because I wasn't certain. The next day, Raymond was off to surgery early in the morning. Everything proceeded according to plan, and soon, Ray was back in his bed convalescing. That evening, his thyroid tests were completed and back on his chart. His thyroid function was zero! The lab had rechecked the result because it was quite literally zero, and the lab had never seen a level that low before. Proudly, I showed the results to the intern, who showed them to the resident, who showed them to the attending surgeon on rounds the following day. Raymond was started on a daily replacement dose of thyroid hormone. A simple and inexpensive solution to a problem that had been overlooked in the past, but that I, a third-year student, had picked up. Raymond returned to the residential center the following day, with instructions to return in two weeks for a final check of the surgical results. He was bandaged but fairly comfortable and actively up and around. At his recheck two weeks later, he was a changed man. Still taking his thyroid replacement, his speech was more normal. He had more energy and had lost some weight, and he told us that he was no longer wearing a sweater. I heard, later on, that he had been discharged from the state hospital and had returned home to live a productive life on the farm with his family. I still ask that same question when doing a complete H& P, but I've never been so lucky as to find someone as treatable as Raymond.

Nurse with Placebo

At a large and busy teaching hospital, a medical student will likely encounter some very strange medical problems. On the internal medical service, as a third-year student, my primary role was to learn to evaluate patients and learn about disease processes. The medical problems encountered at a teaching hospital are often much more complex or rare than those seen in community hospitals. Common things are common, and rare things rare. Teaching hospitals are where rare things are common. It is not unusual for a patient to be referred in for aid in making a difficult diagnosis or when a patient's medications become complex or so numerous that side effects or drug-drug interactions ensue. The teaching hospital is available to help with those difficult situations and make sense of it all.

When a patient enters the hospital, a record is made of that visit, which includes a history of the patient's illness, any symptoms that the illness is producing, and what has been done for that illness, to the current point in time. The past medical history of the patient is also recorded. Any prior hospitalizations, any prior surgical procedures, and any medications taken are all dutifully recorded by the third-year medical clerk. This information is then reviewed and verified by an intern, and likely, an upper-level resident. The patient often grows weary of telling and retelling the same story over and over. Still, it is a process that unveils illness and disease and allows for the development of a treatment plan that is safe and effective.

It was in the midst of this admissions process one day that I learned a great deal about medicine, from an experienced professional. I was admitting a woman in her late sixties to the medical unit for evaluation of some abdominal pain. Her local primary care provider had been unable to make sense of some of her laboratory results and the pain pattern. He wondered if the patient might have problems with her pancreas or other digestive organs and had sent her to the ivory towers for a consultation with the internists there. I went through my well-memorized list of questions, carefully documenting the onset and location of the pain. I probed how the pain had changed over time, whether or not it radiated to other parts of her abdomen, and what she had done at home to treat it. I looked over her lab tests from "outside" and added those to the record. Next, I asked questions about her family history, whether or not specific illnesses ran in her family, and whether or not other family members had similar symptoms. I next documented her social history. She was married, didn't smoke, occasionally drank an alcoholic beverage, but never to extremes, and didn't get much exercise. Finally, I asked her if she took any medications. "Yes," she said, "They are in my suitcase."

I looked over at the bed and saw two suitcases. "I'll need to make a list of them, for the record," I said.

"Bring me the brown suitcase, on the right" was her reply. "I'll get them out for you."

I lifted the rather heavy brown suitcase over onto a chair and helped her open it. She was correct. Her medications were in her suitcase. The whole suitcase was completely full of medicine bottles. I eventually counted over 300 bottles containing 273 different medicines, all legitimately obtained by prescription, in her possession. As we went through the medicines, making note of each medicine, dosing schedule, and when she'd last taken the medicine, I also discovered a small plastic bag of syringes and a bottle of saline. "And this?" I asked, moving along through her lengthy recitation of medicines and their uses.

"Oh," she said, "sometimes I need to give myself a placebo, when the other medicines aren't working." I looked again at my notes and smiled as I reread my record of her social history. Under work history, I had recorded "retired registered nurse." This would be an interesting patient, indeed.

Central Line on Awake Patient

Not all patient dishonesty was as clear-cut; however, there was the time, while I was a third-year student on the medicine service, the team of doctors that cared for nonsurgical patients in the hospital, that a patient really surprised me. We had just received an admission of a patient, in her midsixties, with the diagnosis of stroke. She was transferred to the university hospital for evaluation and treatment of a stroke, which had left her unable to respond and in an apparent coma. She had become unable to speak, did not respond to voiced requests to move her arms or legs, blink, or move her head. She was breathing on her own and had a strong heartbeat, but little else came from her in the way of body functions, including withdrawal from painful stimuli. Doctors and medical students have a variety of ways of determining a person's level of consciousness.

Typically, a person's level of consciousness fits into one of four categories. Either they are alert, awake, and responsive to questioning, or they are drowsy or sleepy and respond only when spoken to, or they are sleepy and only respond to painful stimulus, like a pinch, a pin poke, or a vigorous rub with the knuckles of the examiner on the patient's sternum, or they do not respond to any of these—the truly comatose patient. The patient in question met this last criterion. She lay there, eyes open but unmoving, with no response to verbal, pain, or any other stimulus. I had been asked to help the intern place a central line into one of the major vessels, to provide access to her circulatory system for fluids, and intravenous feedings, until she woke up.

The procedure involved cleaning the skin with a disinfectant, then making a small area of the skin numb, with a local anesthetic, and then inserting a very large hollow intravenous needle into the skin overlying the collarbone. The needle would be guided inward, until it touched the bone, then tilted downward, and inserted further inward, until the tip of the needle passed beneath the lower edge of the collarbone, and at that point, would enter a large vein that is located just under and behind the collarbone—the subclavian vein. Care must be taken because there is also a large artery there, and nerves pass through the area, as well. Most importantly, however, the uppermost tip of the lung is located just beneath these large vessels, and penetration of the lung would likely result in a release of air from the lung, followed by a collapse of the lung. So frequent was this complication that it was standard procedure to get a chest x-ray on every patient after the placement of a subclavian line, to make certain that the lungs remained fully expanded. Dr. M., my intern, was still fairly new and, while he was two years ahead of me in training, he had very little independent experience at that point. This was going to be his first subclavian as an intern. My first one, too, although both of us had seen the procedure done before. He carefully laid out all the equipment and instruments that would be needed for placing the line. We placed the patient into a slightly head-down position, which would help fill up the target vein with blood, making entry into it easier. He put on his sterile gloves and prepared the skin with three quick scrubs with an iodine solution. Then he placed sterile cloth drapes over the collarbone of the patient, leaving a small triangle of bare skin open at the very center of the collarbone. She lay there—unmoving and unresponsive to all that we were doing. Dr. M. was giving me a running verbal description of everything he was doing, reviewing his procedure as much for himself as to teach me. Next, he drew into a syringe a teaspoon or so of local anesthetic. He injected this into the exposed skin, just over the collarbone, creating a small area of numbness. Through this area, he inserted a much larger needle. The needle was sharply pointed, but about as big around as a pencil lead and connected to a syringe. He advanced the needle though the skin, and I saw it bump up against the bone of the collarbone. He tilted the syringe upward, directing the needle downward, and advanced under the collarbone, while drawing back on the syringe to detect the blood that would be visible the moment that he entered into the vein. He aimed the needle's point at the spot where he imagined the upper notch of the breastbone to be, just above the point where the collarbones join it, beneath the chin. Shortly, blood squirted into the barrel of the syringe, indicating the position had been reached. He carefully placed a fingertip over the needle hub while removing the syringe. He threaded a small flexible wire down into the needle and into the vein. This wire would serve as a guide for the large hollow IV line that would follow the wire's course into the vein. He had me make a small nick in the skin, at the point where the wire entered the skin of the chest wall, because the IV catheter is blunt and would not penetrate the skin as the needle had before. Carefully sliding the wire into the hollow center of the IV catheter and advancing the catheter down the wire's length, the catheter progressed along the path to the blood-filled center of the vein. Then it stopped abruptly. He could not advance the tubing any further. He had me try to draw blood back through the hollow catheter, but none would come. Something had gone wrong, and the line could not be placed at that site. We carefully withdrew the tubing and wire and applied pressure over the site to prevent bleeding. We talked about the possible problems and discussed how to best proceed. She still needed the line, and she would be needing volumes of nutrients and medications that would exceed the capacity of IV lines in her hands or arms. We regathered the necessary equipment, and swapped sides. He felt that placing the central line from the patient's other side was the best way to proceed. As I watched from my new vantage point, continuing to hold pressure against the bandage on the site of the previous attempt. He related that he wondered if the prior attempt had failed due to alteration of the normal anatomy by the large dose of local anesthetic injected at the site. He felt that, since she was in a coma, unresponsive to, and apparently unfeeling of pain, he intended to proceed without the anesthetic injection, so as to not disrupt the anatomic relationships beneath the skin. He proceeded the same as before, iodine prep to the skin, sterile drapes, gloves, and then syringe-mounted needle. He penetrated the skin at the midportion of the collarbone, bumped up against it, then maneuvered the needle beneath the edge of the bone. This time, there was no flash of blood into the syringe. He muttered his dismay, then began to move the needle deep beneath the skin, deeper into the subclavian space, looking for the vein. Not finding it, he withdrew the needle, rechecked his surface landmarks, and reentered the skin at a slightly different site. At that very moment, the patient, who had remained absolutely motionless up to that point, slowly turned toward him and said, "That hurts!"

His look of utter shock and surprise was accompanied by a long pause and then, "It does?"

She replied, "Yes, it hurts. It all hurts. Don't do it again." Then she turned back to stare at the ceiling. So much time had passed that I no longer remember the reason for the woman's feigning coma. I do remember that we immediately stopped any further attempts at placing a central line in her and summoned the other members of the team to help in her continued evaluation. I also remember that valuable lesson, though, and to this day, I still always use a local anesthetic on any patient that I do not know, for a fact, is under a general anesthetic. Even then, I sometimes will still inject the site, just to be sure, but I give the excuse that it is to help reduce post-procedure discomfort. I just don't want a patient to turn to me unexpectedly while I'm doing a procedure and tell me that it hurts.

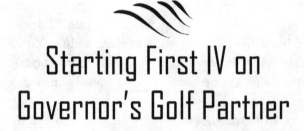

Starting First IV on Governor's Golf Partner

Again, during my third year, I was challenged with another first procedure. Access to an intravenous route into the body is a common method of delivering medications and fluids for hydration. This allows the fluids or medications to rapidly and with certainty become a part of the body's circulatory system and speeds their availability to all the body's organ systems. Therefore, sooner or later, every medical student must place their very first IV line in a human patient. Students usually receive some show-and-tell training prior to their first attempt. This usually involves reviewing the details of the major veins, learning how to choose a good vein, learning what size of IV best fits which situation, how to prepare the skin, how to orient the needle, how to set up the IV fluids, how to puncture the skin, how to recognize the entry into the vein without poking the needle all the way through the vein, and how to secure the IV needle to the arm after success in starting the IV line. For me, the training occurred rapidly on the first morning of my third-year surgery rotation. All surgery patients had IV lines while they occupied a bed on the surgical ward. This included all patients, whether they were awaiting surgery, just completed surgery, or nearly ready to go home. A functioning IV access site was mandatory on all patients, at all times.

On my first day on the surgical team, I made it through rounds pretty much unscathed, with the exception of having been sent to fetch some supplies. By afternoon, I had attended the noon teaching conference and had then gathered with my surgical team to process the incoming patients who were arriving at the hospital with a surgical procedure of some type planned for the following morning. My first patient was a fortyish female who was in good health except for some pesky gallbladder pain and who was planning on having her gallbladder removed by the team the following morning. Let's call her Carol. Now Carol was friendly, talkative, and a bit anxious about her planned surgical procedure. During her H&P, she asked a lot of questions, to which I, as a new surgical student, had few good answers. I could tell that she really wanted someone more knowledgeable to speak to, in order to get the answers she was seeking. However, the procedure was that patients scheduled for surgery would give their history and be examined by a third-year student, followed by an intern, followed by a resident, followed by the chief resident, followed by a review of all of this by the staff surgeon. Because of this way of doing things, patients would actually repeat the same facts over and over, several times. I was certain that the most common question that I heard was "Don't you guys talk to one another? I've told this same story five times!" But, as students, we quickly became used to the repetition, even though the patients didn't. So Carol finished telling me her story, about the pain under her right rib, the nausea after eating, the pain in the nighttime that awakened her from sleep, the intermittent changes in her bowel habits, and the sharp, crampy nature of the pain she had experienced. The next step was to start the intravenous line and draw her preoperative blood work. I had been instructed, and this was to be my first IV start.

I gathered all the necessary supplies and jammed them into the pockets of my still-new, still-white third-year med student jacket. I chose alcohol swabs to clean the skin, half-inch tape to secure the IV once started, a rubber tourniquet, a container of Lactated Ringer's solution with 5% dextrose, a packaged length of plastic intravenous line, and a suitable IV needle. After turning toward the patient's room, I turned back, having second thoughts. I picked up a second IV start needle, just in case I missed the first one. To miss an IV on the first attempt was a common occurrence. Most of the students known to me had suffered that embarrassment at some point. Even seasoned residents missed IV attempts with enough regularity that to do so brought no chiding or ridicule from fellow team members, at all. To miss the second attempt was more rare. Usually only beginners suffered that fate. To miss the third attempt meant that you were crossing the line. Three attempts was the unofficial limit. The unwritten rule was, after three misses, you go get someone else to start the line for you. At that point, it was as much about the level of frustration as it was about the necessary skill. It was felt that, after three misses, you were just too shaky, unprepared, or unlucky to hit it on the fourth try, so turn it over to someone else before you really mess up.

I arrived at Carol's bedside and unloaded the pockets, carefully aligning the required items on the bedside table, going over the checklist in my head—skin prep ready, tape torn into strips, IV container punctured, and line flushed of any air, IV needle ready. I carefully placed the tourniquet around the upper arm, just below the body of the biceps muscle, in order to occlude the veins returning from the hands and lower arms. This would cause the low-pressure blood within the venous system to be held back, creating an increasing pressure within the vein and making the vein puff out, full of blood. With gloved hands, I prepared the skin with the alcohol swabs. I looked carefully at the forearm and hands. Not much in the way of big juicy veins were showing up. Some little tiny blue lines were showing, that's all, not an easy first stick. I patted the back of the hand, as I'd seen others do. This is supposed to mildly traumatize the vein and make it stand out more fully. Still not seeing much. I held the patient's hand down below the side of the bed, hoping that the drop in position would cause the blood to pool in that lowered body part. Finally, I saw a decent vein begin to show through the skin. I uncovered the needle and held traction on the skin. Summoning all the courage I could, I managed to say, "This may poke a bit..." as I touched the needle tip to the skin. I carefully aligned the shaft of the needle with the vein beneath the skin, imagining in my mind that the needle would effortlessly pass through the skin and find its way in to the center (lumen) of the now-bulging vein. The skin was very flexible and pushed along ahead of the needle tip, rather than giving way to the point. Then the needle tip lunged through the skin with a sudden release of skin tension. A dark round bulge began to form beneath the skin right at the point where the needle had penetrated the vein. Dang! I'd missed the attempt by letting the needle pass clear through the vein too quickly, causing leakage around the needle with blood infiltrating the subcutaneous tissue at the site. The only thing to do at that point was to carefully withdraw the needle from the vein and skin and apply pressure to keep the bloody spot from enlarging and bruising.

My confidence was waning, but it was my first attempt on my first IV patient. I still had a second IV needle. The technique that I'd been taught called for me to move to a site higher up the hand or arm. This distal-to-proximal progression of IV attempts ensured that one didn't cause damage to the larger more proximal veins as attempts continued. I loosened the tourniquet in order to allow blood to return to the arm. I carefully checked the location of the veins again, feeling with a fingertip to find a nice, full vein to puncture. I found what I thought was an appropriate vein but by now was a little bit nervous having missed the first try. I continued to make conversation with the patient, apologizing for the missed attempt. She smiled and seemed to take it in stride as I prepped the skin with an alcohol swab, ready to try again. This second attempt resulted in penetration of the skin but not puncturing the vein with the return of blood flow into the catheter. The catheter was designed with a clear plastic hub called the flash chamber that would indicate blood return into the catheter by the presence of red blood in its hollow center. After probing as many times as I dared under the surface of the skin, I noticed that I was starting to create some discomfort in the patient's arm. I held the two-part catheter and withdrew it from the skin, frustrated with my obvious failure at my second attempt.

Because that was my last sterile catheter, I excused myself and left the room to go retrieve some additional supplies. Upon my return, I was happy to see the patient was still smiling and carefully set out my equipment for my third try. Reality was that I also calmed down quite a bit going on my supply search, which I thought would increase my chances of success on my third try.

As I approached the patient's bedside, she looked up at me and said, "Well, if you don't get it this time, I guess I'll have to tell Bob what kind of a hospital he runs here."

I thought to myself, *Bob? The surgeon's name is not Bob. The resident's name is not Bob. I don't even think the administrator's name is Bob.* So like a dummy, I said, "Bob who?"

She smiled at me very wryly and said "Bob Ray, the governor. He golfs regularly at our golf course at home."

Now I was really shaking as I said, "Nothing like putting a little pressure on the med student."

Fortunately, my third attempt, following careful alignment of the IV catheter adjacent to a large juicy vein, resulted in a bright flash of red blood into the catheter hub, followed by a smooth sliding forward into the vein of the catheter needle without further mishap. Both the patient and I were relieved as I reached for the tape, firmly taped the catheter into place, and opened the flow valve to start the IV fluids running. I really would not have wanted her to have to report me to the governor of the state of Iowa.

Always Ready for Anything

A common theme among medical students is that they are at the bottom of the food chain. While serving as a medical student, you are often requested to do the lowly jobs that no one else wants to do. For example, while making rounds on surgery, third-year medical students (M3s) were often sent back to the nurses' station to fetch some needed supply: a bandage, a safety pin, a tube of antibiotic ointment, or something similar. It was something that could have waited, but didn't need to, because there were M3s who could run and get it for the team. Actually, for the resident who requested it, it was because they'd forgotten it in the first place or simply didn't know that they'd need it. But since they'd been an M3 once, themselves, and knew how the system worked, they'd order you to run and get it.

Neal, another med student and I, tired of the repeated trips back to the supply carts, thought we'd try to beat the system, so we began to supply our pockets before rounds, and we began to carry the most-frequently requested items: 4 × 4 pins (four-inch square gauze pads, used as dressings and cleanups), tape, tubes of antibiotic ointment, prescription pads (even though we were not licensed to sign them), and so forth. After a day or two of meeting a request for a 4 × 4 by simply reaching into the pockets of our still-new short-length white coats instead of having to run all the way back to the nurses' station, about one hundred yards, in some instances, Neal and I were feeling pretty proud that we no longer had to leave rounds. I think the residents got together and decided to play the game as well because one morning, while on rounds, the resident got a quirky smile and said, "Davis, get me a red rubber catheter. I'll bet you're not carrying one of those, are you?" Red rubber catheters were long tubes, made of latex rubber and open at one end, with the other end

77

sealed in a point but having side openings to allow fluid to enter without plugging up. They were stretchy, strong, and useful for many things, from serving as a tourniquet for blood drawing to obtaining samples for culture from deep within the far reaches of an abscess to their intended use as a temporary drain for the urinary bladder. I didn't have one in my pocket, and I think he knew that I didn't. I frowned, then headed off down the hall to the supply cart. When I returned, he was still smiling as he took the catheter from me.

The next morning, I had catheters in my pockets, along with several other supplies that might be needed. *I'd be ready this time,* I thought to myself. However, we didn't need any red rubber catheters on rounds that day. Rather, the senior resident requested culture tubes to take a specimen of a patient's wound drainage for lab analysis. This time, Neal had to make the trip. The problem was, there simply wasn't enough pocket space in those jackets to carry one of everything that we might need. When Neal got back to the group with the necessary item, rounds continued. In the meantime, I had to listen to the berating comments about how, just once, it would be nice to make rounds without interruption if those lazy, dumb medical students would just come prepared for rounds.

After rounds, Neal and I hatched a plan. That evening, at home, I helped my wife sew three extra pockets onto the inner lining of the white coat. Big pockets. In addition to the extra pockets in both of our coats, we decided to split up what we carried—no duplicates, so we could carry a larger variety. The next morning, all five pockets bulging on both of our coats, we began rounds. That day, we had it all—catheters, blood tubes, culture equipment, bandaging materials, tape, wraps. No matter what the residents asked for, we provided it, on the spot. After about the fifth or sixth request, the resident noticed the additional pockets on our jackets and burst out laughing. The attending asked what was funny, and he, too, began to laugh. I don't know if he thought we were ingenious or idiots. From that day on, we were known as the packed animals.

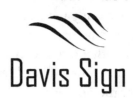

Davis Sign

The second rotation of my third year was general surgery. This rotation generally started early in the morning and often proceeded well into the evening hours except when my team was on call; in which case, we stayed overnight, followed by rounds the next day, and stayed again to the end of the day. This meant that every day I came to the hospital while on surgery rotation, I'd be staying all night that night; however, there was a lot to learn since I was new to any kind of human surgical procedure, having only worked on animals during my research experience. One of the things that happened during the six-week rotation was that I developed a procedure for determining when patients were ready for discharge.

Most of the surgical cases for which I provided care, it seemed, were women patients in their mid- to late forties who are undergoing cholecystectomy for either nonfunctioning gallbladder or the presence of stones within the gallbladder. In modern times, this procedure is carried out through a couple of small incisions in the anterior abdominal wall with the use of a laparoscope. The gallbladders are removed through the scope, which leaves a much shorter healing time and less risk of infection. In the mid- to late seventies, however, cholecystectomy was still carried out through an open laparotomy, which resulted in significant abdominal discomfort through the prolonged healing time. About two weeks into my rotation, I mentioned to our surgery team that I was prepared that day on rounds to predict which patients would be ready for discharge and which might need another day or two before being dischargeable. My senior resident was very interested to hear what I had to say.

Through observation, I had determined that if I walked into a patient's room and found that they were feeling well enough to apply makeup, dress in their underclothing, sit up in bed, and smile, that they were more than likely ready for discharge. This finding seemed to hold true regardless of whether they were ready to take all the medications orally and whether or not they had completely advanced their diet to include regular foods. They literally wore their stage of improvement as a part of their outward countenance. I called this the "Davis positive panty sign," which raised a chuckle from my surgical team. They all saw the rationale present in my description of this sign and were ready to put it to the test. Through the next several days of making rounds, the sign proved itself as being nearly 100 percent reliable and was made into a point of interest by the other surgical teams on the service at that time.

While I don't fancy myself to be on the same level as the physician who described Parkinson's syndrome, McBurney's point, or Collin's sign, it's nice to know that there may be somewhere an eponym based on my name.

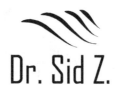

Dr. Sid Z.

The attitude of subservience for medical students was commonly present throughout the surgical service. It had to do, partly, I am certain, with the way that surgeons were trained, at the time. Most surgical training programs, nationally, were what were termed *pyramidal* programs—that is, surgical residencies, predominately five-year-long training programs, took in far more interns into their first years than they graduated at the fifth year. After the first year, a selection was made of the best interns, who were admitted into the second year. The others simply weren't allowed to go on. They had to find training in some field somewhere else. Similarly, after the second year, another selection process led to further narrowing of the number of residents allowed to go on into the third year, and so on. By the fifth year, there were only a handful of spots for training senior residents. The selection process was intensely brutal. You could find yourself having dedicated your time for four years of medical school, and two, three, or four years of residency, and simply have to find training elsewhere. That led to a strict hierarchy, a pecking order whereby, as a medical student, you were lower than low. It also led to an interesting selection process that ultimately led to the production of a surgeon. All that competitiveness bred a certain acidity into their personalities. A part of a common joke that circulated during my medical school years led to the punchline that internists (nonsurgeons) knew everything and did nothing while surgeons knew nothing and did everything. The joke was that pathologists knew everything and did everything, just a little too late to help anyone. So it was, in this training environment, that I found myself learning the healing art of surgery. I spent my first few days in the operating rooms at the university teaching hospital watching the procedures from afar. After all, there was a senior surgery resident who was likely actually doing the case, a junior surgery resident assisting him (or her), and an intern or two scrubbed in to hold retractors (instruments that help hold adjacent tissues out of the surgeon's way so that visibility is ensured throughout the surgical field). Then there would be a scrub nurse to hand instruments to the surgery resident and return them to their place on the table after use. This was all presided over by the attending surgeon—the "boss," one who had vast knowledge of the science of surgery and this procedure and spent the entire operation bringing forth a steady stream of (mostly) pertinent questions.

"What nerve is that?"

"What structure receives blood from that artery?"

"What are two other procedures that would accomplish this same end?"

"What will we be monitoring during the postoperative period?" And, occasionally, punctuating the resident's ignorance with something like "From what embryologic structure did this organ arise?"

Not knowing the answer in these situations was not acceptable. At times, the lack of a correct answer would be met with the stern command "Slide!" after which, positions around the surgical field might change, and someone would be temporarily demoted for some duration. Through this crowd, I spent my first few days watching. Occasionally, one of the surgical team would move aside and let the students actually look at the incision or, even more rarely, peer tentatively into an actual surgical wound, with the wonderful anatomy of the internal parts of the body revealed in all their splendor. After a few days of this type of training, I was finally scheduled for my first actual scrub. I was going to spend the whole morning with my senior resident, the junior resident, and the chairman of the department doing a gallbladder removal. In present times, the gallbladder is usually removed through a small incision by way of a special telescope device that is inserted into the abdomen through an even smaller incision, and the surgical team watches the whole procedure on a TV monitor at the surgical bedside. The surgeon manipulates the scope and a probe or two, along with a specially built knife on a very long handle, and removes the gallbladder through a fairly non-traumatic procedure. But in those ancient days of surgery in the late seventies, the procedure was much more involved. A large incision, eight to ten inches long, was made in the upper right quadrant of the patient's abdominal wall, the underlying tough, fiber layer (fascia) was divided. The underlying muscle layer was cut. The deep fascia was cut, and then the tissue-paper-thin lining layer, the peritoneum, was entered. Then the liver had to be retracted (remember those instruments called retractors held by residents or students?) out of the way, and the gallbladder was located. It was carefully dissected free from its attachment to the liver, and then the duct and artery were clipped with a small metal clip that looked somewhat like a staple. Another clip was placed a short distance away on both the duct and the artery, and then the surgeon would cut between the two clips, which served as seals, so that no liquid leaked out of either end of the severed vessel or duct. The gallbladder was then handed off to the scrub nurse and, from there, off to the observers of the surgery, where the gallbladder sack was opened and, there, before their very eyes, lay the yellow-green gravel or rocks—the gallstones that had been causing the patient's pain. Meanwhile, the duct was carefully checked to see if there were any remaining stones, and then the process of closing the abdomen began. All those layers had to be put back together. Layer by layer, the tissues were brought back together and held by sutures. Stitch by stitch, and all placed carefully by hand. All told, several hundred individual stitches would be required to close an abdominal wound after a gallbladder removal. And I was going to the operating room with both the senior resident and the department chairman. Rumor had been circulating that the department chairman ate medical students for breakfast. At least, it was widely rumored; he yelled at them a lot, a whole lot. Some memories have faded over the intervening years, but I think that the natural adrenalin that was flowing in my veins that morning have helped to permanently imprint some of what transpired.

I recall having read my instruction sheets very carefully and, several times, learning such things as how to scrub my hands using a surgical scrub technique. You have seen the procedure often on television. Each surgeon stands at an individual sink, scrubbing his or her hands with a small soapy brush, for five minutes by the clock. Each finger is individually scrubbed with the soapy pad. The backs, the palms, and then each side of each finger are individually washed, and the nails are scrubbed. Then carefully holding the hands up in the air so that no dirty soap washes down over them and only flows toward the elbows rinses both hands in the stream of water. Turning from the sink still holding the now clean hands in the air, the surgeon walks to the operating room and pushes the door open with a hip, so as to not touch anything with the clean hands. In the operating room, the surgeons are handed sterile towels to use for drying the hands. Carefully the hands, each finger in turn, then the palms, then the wrists, then the forearms, then the elbows are dried. Again, the intent is to not backtrack over clean areas of the arms from dirty areas. Once this process has been completed, the sterile gowns are opened, and the surgeon places his arms into the sleeves, drawing the full-length surgical gowns up over the shoulders. The ties are in the back and are tied by others in the room. A special sterile flap is then extended across the back, which wraps the surgeon in a cocoon of sterile cloth. Lastly, the gloves are placed over the clean hands, drawing them up over the sleeves of the surgical gowns, enclosing the hands, arms, and shoulders in one continuous sterile covering. This last step is many a medical student's downfall. The scrub nurse, already in her sterile gown and gloves, holds the sterile glove open for you. First, your right hand, then your left. The cuffs are folded so that you can pull them on without touching what will become the exposed outer sterile surface of the glove—that is, if you don't reach up with your other hand and touch the glove. However, since you have just washed your hands and you are new to this whole procedure, so you probably didn't know how to thoroughly dry your hands, and since the gloves stick to moist hands, the gloves invariably stick a little, and so you reflexively reach up to help pull the glove onto your hand. The scrub nurse is trained to monitor for any break in sterile technique, and when it occurs, corrects it. In this case, the glove is ripped from your hand, you get a glare and a stern "Don't touch the sterile surfaces!" and you must start the gloving procedure all over again. It only took me three tries to get the gloves on correctly even though I'd read and reread the instruction sheets several times. The thought occurred to me that it was going to be a long day in the operating room. For the opening incision, I was pretty much a spectator, standing off to the side and out of the way. Once the abdominal cavity was entered, however, a retractor was taken from the table and the wide, flattened metal surface, curved to conform to the contours of the internal organs while staying out of the surgeon's way, was carefully placed by the chief resident. He looked at me, only his eyes visible from behind his surgical mask, and handed me the retractor handle.

He commanded me, "Hold this and don't move!"

Now I must admit, after the gloving experience, I was surprised to be entrusted with such an important task. The placement of the retractor, known as a Deep Deaver, was to ensure that the surgeon could see what he was doing, by holding all the other tissue layers out of the way. To be honest, at nonteaching hospitals, there are self-retaining retractors that accomplish this task splendidly, without slipping, growing tired, or having to shift their body weight. At a teaching hospital, however, it was a rite of passage to have to hold a retractor handle, unmoving, and unable to see the far end of the retractor, for most of an hour. But this was my first real surgery, and I was being entrusted with the retractor. I was so excited! Because I had never really done this type of procedure before and because I couldn't really see into the surgical incision, anyway, I was mostly working on holding the retractor very still so as not to move it even the slightest. Despite my best efforts, the senior surgical resident occasionally had to reposition the retractor, telling me, "Stop dancing on the end of that retractor! I can't see!"

The department chief, standing across from us on the other side of the patient, simply kept up his steady stream of questions about the procedure. I was doing pretty well with my answers. My arm was aching from holding it in one position for so long, but I really didn't mind. I was in the operating room. I was "doing surgery." I had seen the insides of bodies before—my cadaver, the brief glimpses during my previous entries into the operating room, but now I was here, on the end of a Deaver retractor, in the operating room.

I saw the gallbladder being handed off in a stainless-steel pan to the scrub nurse. *Ahh*, I thought, *we'll be closing soon, and I can get rid of this stupid retractor.* The surgery resident applied the electrocautery, a device that sends a quick little spark from its tip to seal up small bleeding vessels in the surgical wound. While sealing off bleeding vessels, it also heated the tissues slightly and somewhat "cooked" the blood that was coming from the vessels. The smell was horrendous even through the surgical masks. Next, he asked for the suture material from the scrub nurse. Each suture thread was already placed through the eye of the surgical needle, wrapped around the tip of the needle holder, and handed over in a position that makes it ready to use without having to reposition it. The surgeon then placed the thread into the correct position in the wound and released the thread from the needle. The assistant surgeon, in this case, the head of the department of surgery, then tied the thread, placing several knots, one on top of the previous one until the thread was securely tied. The thread was then cut to a short length, and the next suture was placed. Each suture was placed individually, hand-tied individually, and cut individually. A surgical procedure, such as a gallbladder removal, could take hours, if it were not for the practiced skill that allows the placement of the stitch to be followed immediately by the tying of the knots and then by the cutting of the suture. In a well-practiced operating team, the rhythm that develops allowed the procedure to proceed quickly and smoothly. But then we were not exactly a well-practiced operating team. At least, I wasn't yet. That first day, I thought I'd be done with my part and excused from the operation when I handed my retractor back to the scrub nurse. I was surprised, therefore, when the chief surgeon looked at the senior resident and said, "Should we toss the student a bone and see how well he can cut sutures for me?" Beneath my mask, I was smiling from ear to ear as the scrub nurse handed me a pair of five-inch mayo scissors. My elation soon turned to anguish, however, because as I reached in to cut the first suture, the head of the surgery department turned to me and said sharply, "Too long, make them shorter." I realized that nowhere, in all my reading of the instruction sheets that were to prepare me for this learning experience, had I ever read anything about the proper length to which I should cut the suture material during an operation. I guess I'd never thought about it up until that moment. If the suture is cut too long, excess material remains in the surgical incision after the surgery. That material, foreign to the body, could serve as a source of scarring or lead to an inflammatory reaction or even infection. Yes, each suture is very small, and a short tail on the string wouldn't amount to much, but spread over dozens or even hundreds of sutures imbedded in the surgical wound, it could certainly add up. I'd certainly cut them shorter. The next suture was placed, tied, and then I cut it. Shorter, this time.

"Too short!" came the response. "Do you want them to come untied?" Another glare from behind the mask. I hadn't thought about them coming untied. There were several knots in each stitch. Surely, they wouldn't come untied. I guess they could come untied.

I'd better cut them longer, next time, I thought.

The next several sutures were placed, and each one seemed to be met with either a "too short!" or a "too long!" comment, back and forth. Soon, I got the hang of it, and the warnings became fewer and fewer. The layers were closing, and I was wishing to be out of that room and somewhere else, not having to worry about cutting a suture tail, which I could hardly even see, too short or too long. Finally, after what seemed ages, the deep layers were closed and the surgery resident asked for the "skin suture." I was tired. I was frustrated by not being able to cut the sutures to the right length. I knew that this was likely the end of my career as a surgeon, and that I'd never again be allowed to be entrusted with the scissors to cut the sutures. I'd likely be just a retractor holder from that point on. I'd heard of students that never got the opportunity to do anything in the OR beyond holding a retractor. And here, I'd been given the chance to do something more responsible, and I'd blown it. With the department head, no less. I was doomed.

While frustrated, I heard the chief say, "We're going to close the skin now. Do you think you can cut these sutures to the length that I want them?"

In my frustration, far too quickly, and without thinking, I said, "I think so—do you want them 'too short,' or 'too long?'"

There was dead silence in the operating room. The surgery resident stood there, just looking at me from behind his mask. The scrub nurse stared at me in silence. No one spoke in the OR for what seemed like an eternity. I just stood there, uncertain as to what to do. I couldn't believe that I had said that to the department chairman, Dr. Z., who eats medical students for breakfast. After the longest moments in my life, he began to laugh. The resident then began to laugh, and the scrub nurse began to laugh. Moments later, he composed himself and said to the resident, "Proceed." After the third suture was placed in the skin or so, he turned to me and said quietly, "I want you to write me a well-researched paper on the proper length for cutting sutures. On my desk in four days."

We finished the procedure uneventfully and took the patient to the recovery room, where the resident took me aside and said, "You got off easy—you're lucky to be alive. I can't believe you said that to the chief!"

I wrote the paper, turned it in on time, and successfully passed my surgery rotation.

First Chest Tube

My second rotation of my third year took me to the surgical service. Again, organized into teams, and each team was made up of four third-year students, a fourth-year student, an intern, and several residents. We were on call every other day, and our call included accepting incoming surgical patients as well as covering any surgical problems presented to the emergency department. I've mentioned the importance of procedures to the interest of a medical student. It was what we most looked forward to. It was our payday, making all the long hours and hard work worthwhile. A call to the emergency room was, for a third-year student, the most important thing that could happen. We knew that we'd do little more than observe or hold retractors or cut sutures during an actual operation, so the ER calls were opportunities to actually participate in the care of patients.

One afternoon, my senior resident's pager erupted with a call to the ER, *stat*. As he turned away from what he was doing and broke into a run down the hall, he turned and yelled over his shoulder for me to come along. The surgical wards were on the fifth floor of the hospital and at the opposite end of the building from the ED. The elevators were too slow, so we always took the stairs when running to a call to the ED.

The patient was a man, early forties, who had fallen from the roof of a barn. Most barns in Iowa are thirty to forty feet in height. This farmer had fallen thirty feet onto the muddy barn lot below. His neck was immobilized with a firm plastic collar, and he was strapped to a backboard, but he was having extreme difficulty breathing. His breaths were coming slowly, in gasps, and his color was poor. The resident, Dr. K., listened carefully to his lungs and asked me to do the same. I could hear almost no air movement on either side. A quick exam of his ribs showed multiple broken ribs on both sides, as well. His condition was very poor. Anesthesia was helping us by obtaining a protected airway, but this patient needed both of his lungs re-inflated immediately. This was done by placing a hollow tube through an incision in the chest wall, then sealing against all leaks, and connecting the tube to a low-level vacuum source, drawing the lungs back to their fully-inflated volume.

Here was the drama. Both chest halves were injured, with bilateral collapse of the lungs. Two tubes needed to be inserted quickly. Dr. K. was on one side of the patient, and I was on the other. He looked at me and said, "Have you done this before?" I hesitated for a moment, and he said, "I'll talk you through it."

Now if I had said no, I believed that he would have done both sides himself. If I had said yes, it was my belief that he would have known I was not truthful and would have done both tubes himself. So my smartest move was to say nothing and not force his hand either way.

As the nurses quickly gathered the necessary supplies and instrument trays, he gave me an overview of the procedure. Cleanse the chest wall with iodine solution, numb a large area with local anesthetic, make an incision in the area between the ribs, and extend the incision deep through the muscle of the chest wall, making certain to go *over* the rib and stay close to the top of the rib because the lower edge of the next rib up protects a bundle of blood vessels and nerve that shouldn't be injured. Stay away from the lower edge of the rib—only work with the upper edge of the rib. Poke a finger into the incision to be certain that the lung has fallen away from the incision and won't be harmed. Then insert the hollow chest tube into the incision, using a large curved clamp and directing the tube toward the upper corner of the chest cavity.

I was on the left side, and Dr. K. was on the patient's right side.

I cleaned the skin and scrubbed it with the iodine-soaked 4 × 4 sponges. I drew up the anesthetic and cleared the syringe of air. I injected a large circle of anesthetic around the site, watching closely for what Dr. K. was doing on the other side. I mirrored Dr. K. as he picked up the scalpel and felt the rib surface beneath the skin.

My heart was pounding, and my hand was shaking as I touched the sharp blade to the skin, drawing blood. I firmly pressed into the skin, forcing the scalpel blade deep, until it struck the bone, near the upper edge. I tilted the knife, as I saw Dr. K. finish his incision. I advanced into the intercostal muscle and through the pleura. There was a whoosh of air entering the chest cavity as the underlying lung completely collapsed. I inserted my littlest finger into the incision, feeling the slipperiness of the blood-moistened rib and pleura. I couldn't feel the lung and said so out loud. Dr. K. nodded from his side. He was already picking up the hollow plastic chest tube and clamping it into his surgical instrument, collapsing the tip of the tube between the jaws of the clamp. He briefly showed his finished product to me, then proceeded to insert it into his incision. I fumbled with the tube, fitting it into my clamp and clicking the clamp into a locked, closed position. I had more trouble than Dr. K. because my incision was a little small. Twisting and turning the clamp and tube combination, checking the direction and progress with my finger, I finally popped the pair through my incision and into the hollow chest cavity and released the tube. It slid easily into the full depth of the chest cavity, coming to rest against the opposite wall and bowing a little at the end of travel.

Still shaking, I turned to see the nurse pointing at a large curved needle, treaded with large, black silk suture material. This was the easy part. I'd sutured before and was well practiced. From behind me, Dr. K. said, "Leave long tails as you tie the first knot. The suture thread is used to close the skin around the hollow tube, creating a seal. The long tail threads are then used to wrap around the body of the tube, holding it in place. A couple of gauze pads coated with petroleum jelly are then placed around the tube to complete the air-tight seal."

The nurse then handed me a length of tubing from a sterile package. I connected one end to the chest tube that I'd just inserted, and I handed the other end back to the nurse, who connected it to a water-sealed vacuum outlet. I really couldn't tell much of what was happening at that point, except that some bloody bubbles were coming out of the chest tube on my side and coursing up the vacuum tubing to the water seal, where they collected at the bottom of a plastic chamber.

We got an x-ray at that point, which showed two tubes, placed nearly identically on opposite sides of the chest cavity, and the lung nearly completely re-expanded on both sides.

"Good job, Rookie" was the final statement from Dr. K.

That was how a lot of learning occurred during medical training. "Watch and learn, watch and learn" was the common teaching method employed. As a student, I knew that I had to keep myself open to learning opportunities whenever they occurred. If you weren't willing to try new things, it would have been difficult to learn anything at all.

Waterloo Clinic, Twelve-Year-Old OC'S

During the third-year rotations, which introduce the student to patients through a variety of clinical settings, the student finally begins to evaluate patients independently and even formulate treatment plans, all under very strict supervision, of course. This supervision is generally in the form of residents and interns. So it was, during my third-year rotation in obstetrics and gynecology, that I found myself aboard a small twin-engine airplane, making the two-hour flight to an outlying community, to participate in a gynecology free clinic sponsored by the University Medical School. For their time spent, the students of the university received concentrated and in-depth clinical experiences with a variety of patients (and a variety of health-care needs) that was, being based in community setting, much different from the patient base within the hospital. Because I had plans to practice in a community setting rather than a university-teaching-hospital setting, I eagerly volunteered for as many of these outreach clinics as I could. This particular clinic carried the reputation as being strongly inner city in character. The city wherein the clinic was held was known as having a strong work ethic and low unemployment, but enough low income and poverty to generate strong interest in a free clinic.

These clinics actually drew patients with a variety of complaints, but as M3s, we were pretty much relegated to contraceptive exams: performing pelvic exams and pap smears toward the goal of renewing the patient's prescription oral contraceptives. The residents were the recipients of all the interesting patient complaints into their schedule. Oh, occasionally, a student would pick up a cervical erosion, vaginal infection, or imagine a lump in the area of the tube or ovary. But because of the use of the pill, not many ovarian cysts (the pill actually helps in prevention of cyst formation) or uterine tumors (being within the childbearing years, the patients mostly were too young to have this problem yet).

The clinic population was heavily slanted toward minority demographics but contained a sprinkling here and there of Caucasians. One of my patients that day was remarkable and memorable in a variety of ways. I was working my way through a fairly long schedule of twenty-somethings, all requesting renewal of their contraceptive prescriptions. I had developed a routine of beginning the next patient's visit—introducing myself, checking the history and demographics, and then leaving the room for the patient to change into the exam gown and the nurse to set up the room for the exam, then returning to the prior patient's room to write the prescription, deliver the instructions, and check for any last questions, then returning to the next patient's room to complete the exam and pap test. This way, I could use two rooms, bouncing back and forth, and move more efficiently through the schedule. I was starting a new patient then; when holding the chart in my hand and entering the exam room, I was struck by the patient's appearance. She was very young. She had blond hair and pale skin and appeared to be in her early teens, a strikingly different specimen than the other women on my patient list so far that morning. She was clean and neat, but not fashionably dressed. I quickly looked at her chart—she was twelve years old. My immediate thought was *Finally...something interesting...probably.* I thought that she was here for questions of delayed menarche, pelvic pain, or some other noncustomary complaint. I checked her forms. Under the Complaint heading was the same phrase I'd been seeing in that location all morning: *contraceptive counseling.*

"You are here for the pill?" I asked, with what must have been some surprise in my voice.

Yes was her quiet reply.

I mustered my most unassuming and nonjudgmental voice to produce the words "Are you sexually active?"

She replied, again, in a quiet voice, "No."

I continued, "Then why would you want to start the pill?"

She replied, "I don't want to get pregnant."

I have to admit that, at least once, the thought crossed my mind that she probably didn't know how to get pregnant. I paused, thinking of whether or not to discuss the topic further, get some experienced assistance, or simply proceed with the requested exam. In Iowa at that time, minors could request contraceptive information and counseling without parental permission, due to recently passed legislation. For a variety of reasons, however, I usually discussed the topic of parental knowledge with minors because I felt that it was inevitable that the parents would learn of the minor's actions, and I wanted the patient to be prepared to have that conversation with her parents at some future time. Contraceptive pill packages were not small and were not easily secluded. More than once, I had dealt with situations where "Mom found out." As I moved across the room toward the examination equipment, I casually asked, "How do you think your mother will react when she learns of your decision?"

She immediately answered, "She's in the waiting room. She's the one who sent me in here."

After further discussion with the patient, I learned that she really wanted her mother to be present for the exam, but clinic guidelines didn't allow visitors during the exams. Only the patient, doctor(s) and the nurse/chaperone were allowed.

I persuaded the nurse to make an exception and brought the patient's mom in. She was in her midtwenties, having entered motherhood also as an early teen. In the waiting room, I met the grandmother, who was in her late thirties. With two generations of early teen pregnancy in this family, I could then understand their desire for early intervention and prevention for this next generation. I couldn't help but think that it might have been equally effective to have discussed the cause, as well as the treatment for this early fecundity. That said, she received the requested exam and prescription. She left with her mom and grandmother, happily chatting about some topic of interest as they exited through the automatic double glass doors of the clinic.

I certainly learned a lot during that clinic session. Although I attended two more similar clinics in that same community, I never saw that patient again, but I think of her situation nearly every time I hear of a school district debating sex education or see an article on teen pregnancy rates.

Surgery "Night-Light"

Students and residents at the University of Iowa were provided with an on-call room that they stay in when they required to be at the hospital overnight. Most times, as third- and fourth-year students, we were busy enough that we did never see the inside of the call room but rather spent our time in the nurses' station either working out or discussing cases. I was on call on the surgery service one evening when I was approached by my surgical intern who said she had a problem and wondered if I could help her solve it. She said the night-light in the on-call room was not working and was seeking my advice for a solution to the problem.

The on-call room was physically separated from the surgical ward and located on a different floor. I accompanied my surgical intern, Dr. K., to the on-call room, anxious to be of assistance. The nightlight, as it turned out, was just an x-ray view box mounted to the wall that when turned on provided adequate light in the darkened room so that you didn't bump into things if you are awakened in the night for an emergency call. Dr. K. pointed at the light and said, "I don't know why it stopped working. It just won't light up anymore." Being a naive and an inexperienced farm boy, it didn't occur to me that she might have an ulterior motive. I flipped the switch on and off and found that the light box was indeed not functioning. It was plugged in, and so I carefully inspected the view box and saw that it had a Plexiglas surface that would just slide to the side and could be removed. I did this in order to look inside of the view box and saw that the fluorescent tubes were slightly out of position and were no longer making electrical contact with the fluorescent socket. I gave them a quarter turn and was rewarded by the flickering return of the light output within the darkened room. I felt very proud of myself for having solved the problem and turned to Dr. K., expecting accolades for the simple fix to the troublesome night-light. As I turned, I saw that she seemed rather disappointed despite the return "of the outflow of the light."

"Well, it looks like that's got it fixed," I said cheerfully and turned toward the door in order to leave. I didn't realize how native I was until I heard her say, "Aren't you going to stay? That's how I got through my junior clerkship."

I hurried toward the door, and as I reached the handle, I turned and said, "Well, that's not how I plan to get through my clerkship." I opened the door and rapidly exited. As I took the stairs back to the surgical ward, I remember being perplexed about what it just occurred. I wasn't sufficiently familiar with gender harassment, and I wasn't self-assured enough with my place on the surgical team to report it to any senior personnel. That was my one and only brush with what would be later known as sexual harassment, but I later learned from some of my classmates that they had experienced similar requests from a variety of individuals. Other than a few flirtatious comments from junior and senior residents, I was not aware of any ongoing harassment generally in my university training program. As an afterthought, I realized that surgeons often have a reputation and notoriety for being difficult to work with, and I wondered sometimes if the pyramidal nature of their training program wasn't somewhat responsible for this outcome. The Brown program was very competitive the general surgery program was very competitive with fewer resident openings in the subsequent years, causing heavy competition for the remaining spots each year. I ended up passing surgery as a rotation and didn't hear another comment about this experience from Dr. K.

Open-Heart Debut

During my third-year surgery rotation, I was selected from among other students to do a special two-week rotation in the subspecialty area of thoracic surgery. This was in no small part due to my friendship with one of the thoracic surgeons. This was a strange and unknown area to me, and although I was doing well in my surgery rotation, in general, I found that I was totally unprepared for the first open-heart surgery that I was scheduled to observe. Open-heart surgery uses a full surgical team with extra personnel, including extra nursing staff, a pump technician, a surgeon, and three assistants. My position as observer was to be at the head of the bed with the anesthesiologist behind the ether screen watching the surgery. I wasn't required to scrub, so I simply watched as they set up the room and asked questions about their activities and job assignments. As the surgery case started, I was most interested in the bypass pump, watching the pump technician prime the pump with whole blood and crystalloid solution. I really hadn't turned my attention much to what the surgeon was doing until I heard the buzzing of the cautery indicating the entry into the chest cavity. At this time, I stepped up closer to the anesthesia screen in order to see the focus of their attention. I saw the bone saw as it divided the sternum, exposing the heart and pericardial sac. I still remember the sights and sounds of that experience. When I was a teenager, I had had experience with cadavers and had observed many autopsies because of my father's professional capacity. I thought I was pretty well prepared to deal with my experience. I remember the coiled blood tubing being handed off to the scrub nurse and then watched as the tubing filled with bright red blood as it traveled to and from the cardiac bypass pump.

In a very short time, the surgeon turned his head to see how I was doing and said to me, "You need to sit down." I mumbled that I think I need to go to the bathroom and excused myself from the room. I hate to say it, but I got very dizzy and lightheaded and had to sit down in the hallway outside the operating room until my near syncope past. The only other time in my professional career that I didn't do well with sights and sounds of my profession was during my senior rotation when I observed my first case undergoing electro-shock therapy for a patient with severe depression, and later when, as a resident, I had to identify the remains of a severely burned infant in a rural emergency department. I learned that I have a pretty strong stomach although it was not invincible. These experiences, however, prepared me greatly for the things that I would see and do later on as a practicing physician in the area of emergency medicine.

Anesthesia / Surgery Turf Wars

The world of surgery was an eye-opener for me, and I learned a lot on that rotation. I learned about surgeons' egos and how they could take control in the operating room. While this was most often an important safety principle for the benefit of patients and staff, it could be somewhat difficult as well. One such example was a situation I witnessed one afternoon during a vascular surgery case. The surgeon planned for a procedure to remove calcified lining of the carotid artery in an effort to help prevent future strokes for this patient. This required putting a pressure monitor catheter into the carotid artery for obtaining measurements of the internal pressure. The procedure called for the surgeon to take a sterile catheter and hand the end of it to the anesthesiologist who would then connect up to the pressure monitor at the head of the patient. Because the catheter started out sterile, but the end once handled by the anesthesiologist would no longer be sterile, this required a proper procedure for passing from one physician to the other in order to maintain sterility. Now it was commonplace during a surgery to have interactions between sterile and nonsterile personnel, and this usually proceeds without incident and in a cooperative manner. This particular case however was marked by a relatively stubborn anesthesiologist and an equally stubborn surgeon. At the time that the catheter should've been passed from one physician to another, that second physician was not ready to receive the handoff and resulted in the catheter falling across the anesthesia screen, missing the anesthesiologist's hands. All this really meant was that the anesthesiologist had to reach out and pick up the loose catheter and plug it into the monitor. What resulted instead was a very unprofessional exchange between the anesthesiologist and the surgeon with the anesthesiologist eventually refusing to connect the catheter tip to the monitor for the surgeon. This caused tempers to quickly flare, and I witnessed the rise in the situation from a verbal altercation to include the threats of the exchange of blows. All the surgical team present stood uncomfortably by as the two strong personalities faced each other down across the anesthesia screen. I really thought they were going to strike each other.

The case was delayed then for a few minutes while the two exchanged threats and words in a very unprofessional way. Eventually, the connection was made, and the case proceeded in relative silence because of the two strong personalities that were no longer speaking to each other. In a way, I was sorry to witness this unprofessional behavior but also developed a lot of respect for the process of collegiality, working together, and accepting the shortcomings of others. I recall this case in particular not only because of the unprofessional exchange that occurred but because this case fell on the day of my final exam in surgery, which was a written exam. The case was a very long case, and so I had to break scrub to leave the operating room in the middle of the case to go take my final exam. I finished the exam and returned back to the operating room to find about two hours had passed, and he was still performing the same case on the same patient. I rescrubbed my hands, reentered the operating room, received new gown and gloves, and took my place among the surgery team. There was no prolongation of the case because of the temper tantrums of the two physicians, and no complications occurred as a result of that.

Open-Heart Surgery, Closing Leg

During the two-week special rotation and cardiothoracic surgery, I had the opportunity to scrub in on several open-heart surgeries after that first one. There were a couple of reasons for this. First, a good friend of mine was on the thoracic surgery faculty, and because I knew him from church, we were pretty good friends, and in fact, as my surgical experience increased, he used to call me on weekends or evenings when he needed an extra set of hands in the operating room. Due to this connection, my actual surgical experience was much greater than it would have been from just medical school alone. Due to his influence, I had the opportunity to work on many pediatric cases of open-heart surgery and witness firsthand the delicate process of working on very small hearts. Also, due to my previous research experience, he had called me to the operating room on two or three previous occasions, to obtain specimens of cardiac muscle that he was removing so that I could examine it using electron microscopy. This was usually during a case for a disease called IHSS, which is where the aortic outlet muscle thickens and blocks the outlet to the heart. We were trying to determine a process by which this enlargement occurred because it was related to our research in cardiac hypertrophy. I really enjoyed these extracurricular trips to the OR, and it enabled me to expand on my knowledge beyond the experience of the typical student. One direct result of this more frequent experience in the operating room was that I was granted a few extra opportunities. One such memorable opportunity occurred several times during a procedure that was being performed regularly at the university hospital, that of cardiac bypass.

During bypass surgery, which is generally done on older patients when their arteries become blocked by calcium hardening of the arteries, portions of a leg vein (saphenous vein graft) are moved to be used to bypass the area of blockage. In order to do this procedure, first, the saphenous vein is harvested from the patient's leg, which requires a very long incision, approximately fifteen to twenty-five centimeters in length. This vein is then divided into shorter pieces and is then transferred into the chest where it is first attached to a small opening made in the aorta and then placed alongside the heart to a point near the surface where coronary artery can be found that is blocked. A small opening is made in the coronary artery, and the vein is grafted in such a way that connects the blood supply from the aorta to the blocked area of the coronary artery, bypassing the blockage.

My part in this procedure involved assisting with the placement of the patient on bypass and then concentrating my attention on closing up the long laceration that had been made in the leg. In all honesty, I was fairly slow at suturing, and it took me almost as long to close up the leg laceration as it did for the other surgeons on the team to place three, four, or five bypass grafts. Through this process, I became quite adept at closing skin, and this experience aided me greatly in my future professional activities. It became very easy for me to place sutures close together and under no tension, which are the requirements for a good plastic closure. In fact, the surgeon commented a couple of times that I probably should work harder at leaving the patient a bigger scar so that the patient had something to show as a result of the surgery. This suturing experience also proved itself to be very valuable in my future work in emergency departments of various hospitals.

As a result of this additional access to suturing experience, by the time I was in my fourth year and was working at my emergency room rotation, I was experienced enough to close facial lacerations on my own with only cursory supervision. I do recall that the first time I sutured the patient's face, it came on the case of a middle-aged carnival worker who had been involved in a fight that had left him with a large laceration of his for head and cheek. Noteworthy comment by the attending physician was "Well, it's probably impossible to make him look any worse" because of the previous scarred areas present all over his face. I do think that mine turned out better than any of the others.

The other unintended consequence of all this early open-heart experience was that later on, when my own aortic valve began to close, due to scarring, it was recommended that I have an aortic valve replacement. This prior open-heart experience gave me direct knowledge as to the procedure and potential complications that could occur. Although nearly twenty-five years had passed in the interim, when the anesthesiologist asked me if I had any questions preoperatively, I was able to say and be completely sure that I, indeed, did not have any questions at that time.

"No, I know the procedure, and I know you're going to hurt me."

One other memorable event occurred during that two weeks of cardiothoracic surgery. I was scrubbing for an early-morning case as part of the surgical team, and I finished scrubbing my hands and had entered the operating suite in order to receive my gown and gloves preparatory to surgery. The circulating nurse was busy unpacking instruments. The pump technician was sitting next to the pump console filling the tubing with fluids for the upcoming circulatory bypass. The anesthesiologist was in place at the anesthesia screen, and the scrub nurse was helping the surgeons don their gowns and gloves, which was part of the standard daily routine. What occurred next was amazing and made a lasting impression on me to this day. The surgeon for the case was standing face-to-face with the scrub nurse, had his arms outstretched in order to receive the sleeves of his gown, to be followed by his gloves. At some point along in this process, the surgeon for some reason noticed redness in the scrub nurse's eyes and detected a small sniffle emanating from her. He stopped the gowning and gloving process right there and asked her what was wrong. She replied words to the effect that it was nothing, no big deal, and continued to hold his gown out for him to enter his arms into the sleeves. He then stopped and said, "No, tell me what is wrong." Now I was standing in line, third or fourth back to be gowned, and didn't even catch on to the nurse being upset. What I learned was that the nurse had been scheduled to have vacation from the department for her upcoming wedding three days hence and had just learned from the department that her vacation had been canceled due to conflicts in the schedule. I recall the surgeon shaking his head saying, "No, I can't operate when my surgical team is not happy." He then proceeded to break scrub, leave the operating suite, go to the office of the director of nursing, and successfully requested that his nurse be granted her time off for a planned and scheduled wedding. He returned to the operating room, rescrubbed his hands, regowned, and then proceeded with the planned surgical procedure.

What was impressive with this experience was the care that this surgeon had for his coworkers and team. I tried to remember this lesson several times over the ensuing years to be certain that I watched out for the needs of my team and tried to stay tuned to the moods in the operating room and others on the staff who worked with me. Many years later, I was attending a meeting sponsored by insurers of our malpractice policies where they were talking about ways to avoid malpractice claims. The speaker at that meeting likened the surgical process to that of an aircraft carrier launching costly aircraft. The point of the talk was "Who has the ability, on an aircraft carrier, to cancel the launching of an aircraft?" The answer was, surprisingly, that anybody on the aircraft carrier has the ability, and indeed the responsibility to cancel a planned launch if a dangerous situation arises that should prevent such a launch. Too many times, I learned, people have information at their disposal, which they are afraid to act upon, but which would dramatically increase the safety and efficacy of our health-care system. Contrast this with what I've already said about the disagreements between a different type of surgeon personality and the anesthesiologist in control of the case. No similarity, whatsoever.

Dermatology Clinic's Dr. Sample

One of the more fun rotations during my third year was a short two-week rotation in dermatology. There was not a lot of pressure on this rotation, and the dermatologist had a reputation for not being the hardest workers in the hospital. This was an opportunity to learn a lot about skin diseases, although most of them were not very serious or dangerous and almost no emergency cases. One of the required activities was to staff the dermatology clinic on a daily basis. Because so much in the area of skin disease involves visual identification, the clinic had a practice of notifying all students on the service at the time of the presence of an interesting case by calling "Dr. Sample" on the overhead paging system in the clinic. Whenever the Dr. Sample call came out overhead, all the students present would stop by the room to see the interesting case. One afternoon, I was working my way through a series of schedule clinic drop-in visits, when I found my next patient to be a very attractive young college coed who come by the term clinic because she had a rash for four days that hadn't gotten better, and she had not been able to identify the cause. Without paying much attention, I handed her a gown and said, "Please put this on, leaving the rash uncovered."

I exited the room and waited a few minutes for her to change clothing. I walked back into the room and found her, to my surprise, sitting on the exam table, holding the gown in her lap, stark naked. I could feel my face immediately flush, due to embarrassment. I stammered, "I…I…wanted…you to put the gown on."

She replied, "You said to uncover the rash, and it's all over my body."

I grabbed a sheet and handed it to her to hide under and went out to contact the supervising dermatology resident and simply said, "I think I've got a good Dr. Sample case."

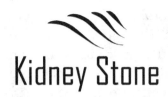

Kidney Stone

It is probably inevitable that all physicians will eventually become ill in some way. In fact, I knew many medical students and residents who had chosen their current area of study or their life's profession because of some close or personal experience with a particular branch of medicine. For example, I knew of an orthopedic surgeon who had a permanent deformity in his upper leg, which caused him to walk with a bit of a limp. Other orthopedic surgeons that I knew had been avid sports participants and had chosen orthopedics for its close alliance with sports injuries. It seemed that most ophthalmologists wore glasses, and most psychiatrists needed one. For me, this personal experience was leading me toward a career in family medicine, the evolved form of the general practitioner of previous times. It was nearly sidetracked, however, during my fourth year when I became the patient. I always thought myself to be in good health, athletic as a youth, a collegiate football player, although, admittedly, I'd given most of my time to studies and other responsibilities and had greatly slackened, er, uh, nearly eliminated my workout schedule. Still, I considered myself invincible, though a little soft. I could still bike to school with little more than a little puffing on the hills. I had just finished my dermatology rotation, where I'd taken up the game of racquetball, and had moved on to a term on the pediatrics inpatient unit. It seemed that dermatology residents had enough free time in their schedule that they were able to take long lunches, with a game or two on the courts before returning to afternoon clinics, and I'd picked up the habit. Even though I now had less time and a busier schedule on pediatrics, the sports field house was adjacent to the medical school and hospital, and I could hear the squash and racquetball courts calling my name every afternoon from across the parking lot. I indulged myself, convincingly reminded that I needed the exercise. I had just finished playing a quick game and headed to the shower for a quick clean up when I stopped by to empty my bladder. I don't remember anything unusual during the game or beforehand; only afterward when, upon looking down at the progress of the urine stream, I noticed that it was a dark-burgundy color. My urine was bloody! I quickly thought back to the game I'd just played and didn't recall any trauma, falls, or bumps. I didn't hurt anywhere, and it wasn't even uncomfortable now. My current level of medical knowledge didn't take me far enough into the functioning of the urogenital system to know what else might cause such a thing to occur. After I finished, I mentioned my observations to my classmate. We agreed that I should go to the urology clinic to see what might be causing the blood. I found the urology clinic easily on the hospital's fourth floor. I was in luck that one of the current interns in the clinic that afternoon was one of my prior surgery interns. As soon as I explained my symptoms, he said, "Kidney stone," as if pronouncing my sentence to death.

"But I don't have any pain," I said, demonstrating again my limited knowledge and lack of experience in the area of urology. I had already served my brief two-week rotation in urology, as a junior student, rescuing, as I did, a man from the state mental hospital, but I had never seen anyone with a kidney stone during the whole two weeks on the service.

Kidney stones are actually relatively common, as I was to learn, but due to their frequency, they are usually treated in the community hospitals and rarely make it to the medical mecca of a teaching hospital. Unless they walk in, of course, as I had just done. I had to generate a specimen of urine for analysis, something that was easier to request than to supply, given that I had just emptied my bladder trying to see if the blood would stop. Yes, all that burgundy color was due to red blood cells in my urine. No infection, at all, just blood. I was asked about pain (none now, none ever), about having had previous stones (none), and about my health history. Not much to report, just that I'd had my tonsils out at age five, because my sister had frequent sore throats, and was getting hers out, and the doctor had said, "Have them both in the hospital in the morning." Otherwise, the only time I'd seen a doctor was to have some sutures in my elbow after falling during a track meet while trying to pass a baton to a fresh runner during a relay event.

I was then sent to put on a gown and taken to the x-ray room. I had an IV started, and a plain x-ray of my abdomen taken, from my ribs down to my hips. There it was, on my right side, high up near my kidney, a round white spot that was indicative of a calcium-containing stone in my kidney collecting system. Next, they injected some contrast material into my veins and took several more radiographs in rapid sequence, watching the contrast course through my kidneys, being excreted into the urine, and causing the kidneys, collection plumbing, and drain tubes to light up. I say contrast out of habit, having learned that to be the proper term the previous year while on the urology service. If a student or resident were to ever mistakenly refer to that substance as *dye*, one of the attending urologists was well-known for chastising you on the spot, walking around, shaking his head, and waving his arms while saying in a very loud and condescending voice, "Dye? Dye? That is not dye, Doctor. That material is contrast. Patients die. Kidneys get contrast." In fact, he became so well known for repeating this statement that during the annual senior skit later that year, the offending urologist was lampooned during a presentation of a spoofed patient wherein at the end of the case recital, the reporting "doctor" confirmed the patient's unfortunate demise by declaring, "Despite all our best efforts, the patient contrasted."

The stone was about a centimeter across, just under a half inch, which is large by kidney-stone standards, and likely too big to pass on its own. This was before the newer methods of treating such stones came into being. Now a stone of that size would be subjected to a focused shock wave of sound energy, which would be expected to shatter the stone, breaking it into multiple small and passable fragments. The process called lithotripsy eliminates the need for an open surgical procedure in most cases, but as I said, it hadn't been invented yet. I set up a consultation with the attending urologist. It was his opinion that I hadn't had any pain yet because the stone was too large to pass into the tubing. When a stone enters the ureter, the tube that connects the kidney with the bladder, the muscular ureter may constrict, causing spasmodic pain in the flank and back or around into the front of the abdomen, groin, thigh, or even seem to hurt into the testicle. I'd had no such pain, so the assumption was that the stone had not or could not pass into the ureter. I was about four weeks from my senior interview trip. During this trip, I would travel to various residencies and interview for a position in their program. I didn't want to interfere with that trip, and besides, I wasn't even hurting, and I wasn't losing blood rapidly enough to be significant. The attending urologist felt that a period of simply watchful waiting would be acceptable, but he cautioned me that if the stone became infected, or if I started to have pain, more immediate attention would be required. Over the next three or four hours, the blood cleared up and didn't return. In the meantime, I was going to my pediatrics rotation each day, making rounds, doing admission workups on ill children, and hoping that nothing happened before my interview trip.

Pediatrics at a teaching hospital was not at all what I'd anticipated. Instead of seeing and learning about young folks with pneumonia, earaches, or other common illness that typically afflict children, those were taken care of in the outlying community hospitals, and the university teaching hospital received mostly the complicated, rare, and challenging cases that were referred in. This process, known as "herding the zebras" comes about because common childhood illnesses are, well, common. They are the equivalent of horses in the equine world, being seen frequently and recognizable and treatable by most doctors. Other illnesses, either by virtue of their rarity or because they are unresponsive to usual treatments, perhaps even untreatable, are known as "zebras," and the comparison has led to a commonly uttered adage about illness that says, "When you hear hoofbeats, think of horses but look for zebras."

My pediatrics unit was a herd of zebras. There were some children being evaluated for complex birth defects, a couple of brittle diabetics who were admitted for aid in controlling their blood-sugar levels, and a particularly unfortunate young man with childhood leukemia who was admitted for chemotherapy. I was responsible for delivering his chemotherapy through multiple-times-per-week injections of methotrexate, a potent chemical poison, directly into the fluid around his spinal cord. This was a very uncomfortable procedure that required that the child/patient receive an injection of local anesthetic into his back, followed by the introduction of a three-inch long spinal needle into the sac of fluid that surrounds the spinal cord with the withdrawal of a small amount of fluid and the replacement of the lost fluid with the chemotherapy. Finally, the child had to lie recumbent for a few hours after the treatment session, ensuring that the fluid didn't leak out. This procedure was repeated every other day, for three weeks. I inherited this patient when I came onto the service midway through the boy's chemotherapy course. For me, the process gave me many opportunities to perform lumbar punctures. I couldn't help, however, feeling great empathy for the patient, watching him try to prepare himself and watching him try to endure the procedure time after time. He was actually a very brave young man, suffering through my inexpert technique in mostly good spirits. We developed a close relationship, him teaching me to refine my technique into a painless puncture on the first pass each time, and me spending some of my time on the service playing board games or other pastimes to help alleviate the boredom of spending a large part of your childhood in a hospital.

It was the fall, and Halloween was rapidly approaching, falling on a Saturday that year. I had secretly made plans with several of the nurses' stations located close to the pediatrics unit to have treats available on Halloween so that the med students could take some of the more mobile patients around for some trick-or-treating. I was planning to borrow some surgical scrubs, a mask, and a surgical hat and dress up my patient as a doctor. Not very original, I agree, but easily done with the materials at hand. I mentioned it to him a couple of days before, just to be certain that he would be available, and he was very excited at the prospect.

Thursday, two nights before Halloween, I was home, studying. All of a sudden, I felt a deep ache in my right lower chest, along my back ribs. It immediately took my breath away. Within a few seconds, I was sweating, in extreme pain, bent over, unable to stand up straight. The pain was unlike any I'd ever experienced. I could hardly speak and headed immediately to the bathroom, in the midst of a wave of nausea flooding my brain. My wife came to check on me, worriedly trying to help me. Unfortunately, there were very few things that help the pain of renal colic. After about thirty minutes, I was convinced that I was going to die, and afraid that I wouldn't. My wife loaded me into the car, quickly made arrangements for a sitter for the kids with one of the neighbors, and drove me to the hospital emergency room. I walked in slowly, still bent over, pale and sweaty, and hovering over a large plastic bowl.

"Kidney stone," I said to the resident on duty. "I need something for the pain."

Many years of experience have taught me that kidney stone patients frequently present to the emergency department in just this very way. Whether due to pride or bravado on the part of the patient, which leads them to believe that they can "wait it out" and avoid the expense and inconvenience of a trip to the ED, or simply due to the inability to get themselves to the ED, many stone patients arrive at the ED well-engaged in the severe pain that can accompany a stone passing. Still, it is not uncommon for those who are actually seeking recreational narcotics, or a *fix* for a well-established drug habit, to present to an ED feigning a kidney stone. Some will even go so far as prick a finger in the privacy of a restroom while obtaining the required urine sample, in order to get a drop or two of blood to add to the urine to make their complaint seem more plausible. No wonder that this experienced resident didn't immediately reach for the syringe on the basis of my request alone.

"What makes you think you've got a stone?" he asked.

"I've had x-rays upstairs in urology last week," I explained. "I've got a centimeter-wide rock sitting in my right ampulla," I added, trying to sound both knowledgeable and authoritative despite my desire to puke everything out from my toes to my head.

"Any blood in your urine?" was the next question.

"Not today, but last week my pee was a perfect burgundy color after a racquetball game," I said, mistakenly adding an unneeded distraction to the resident, who was my ticket to pain relief.

"Did you have any trauma before the blood?" he asked, taking the unintended bait and adding traumatic kidney injury to his differential diagnosis list.

"No trauma, just the blood, then the IVP, which showed the stone. Everything else was normal," I said, trying to get him back on track toward administering some analgesic.

"Sure, sure," he said, not moving from his position.

I must admit that I recall that time clearly. Oh, the exact feeling of the pain could no longer be summoned to mind, and I've had other painful experiences since, which come close to or surpass those moments. However, enough of my wicked thoughts and malevolence toward that resident's delay remain imprinted in my mind that I almost always get the nurse moving toward the delivery of pain medication to kidney stone patients while I remain behind to finish my history-taking and physical evaluation. I always place analgesic as a top priority for renal colic, preferring to err on the side of giving unneeded medication to withholding desired relief to the patient. I'm nothing if not educable.

So finally, after what seemed an eternity of questions, the requested films appeared from urology, and the diagnosis was confirmed. I got an IV, and my first dose of pain medication. I'd never experienced narcotics before, and I remember the strange feeling that came over me when the nurse pushed the medication into my IV line. I thought to myself, *Why do people pay big money to feel this way?* I recall that I felt like my head was getting cloudy, and I noticed that I couldn't talk very well, but my pain was still there—every bit of it. The dose was repeated. Then it was repeated a second time. The resident commented that I was requiring enough pain medication that he was concerned that I might stop breathing.

"That would be okay with me," I think I said, meaning that at least the pain would stop. I went through the admission process, filling out and signing papers, with my wife's assistance. I would be admitted for twenty-four hours, to see if the stone would move at all. If not, I would need to have the stone surgically removed. It was apparently too large to crush or to remove "from below" by passing an instrument up through my urethra, bladder, and lower ureter. My pain was intense, and just before taking me upstairs to my room on the elevator, they gave me another dose of analgesic medicine. In the elevator, the resident said that he hadn't seen a stone that large before. My reply was to vomit on his shoes in the closed confines of the elevator. The next eighteen or so hours were a blur of pain and narcotic-induced semiconsciousness. I had an IV in my arm, both as a route for the medication and as a source of needed fluids since I was too nauseous to keep anything down. Finally, the pain let up a bit, and I was able to go a while without medication and get up for short walks, hauling my IV pole along with me.

The following day, a repeat x-ray showed that my stone had not moved a bit. The consulting urologic surgeon thought that my stone was too big to pass, sitting instead in the funnel-shaped collecting system of my right kidney, occasionally sliding into the neck of the funnel, blocking the flow of the urine and producing the severe pain. Occasionally, the stone would dislodge and slip into the wider part of the funnel, allowing the urine to pass and relieving the pain. The stone was acting as a sort of ball-valve, intermittently blocking my urine drainage system. I was going to need surgery, and I was put on the schedule for Sunday morning.

Saturday was a pretty good day, with some episodes of pain in the morning. Afternoon, though, was pretty quiet. By late afternoon, my head was clearing from all the medication earlier in the day, and I suddenly remembered my planned rendezvous with the costumed treat solicitor. I convinced my nurse that I'd be okay for the trip down two floors and halfway down the length of the hospital to the pediatrics ward to take my young charge around to receive his candy, but I'd have to go as I was, IV and all.

As I slowly made my way up to the nurses' station on pediatrics, my gown carefully tied in the back to minimize my exposure to the world and pulling my IV bag, attached to a rolling IV pole along beside me, there sat my patient, already dressed in the green scrub clothes of a budding surgeon, mask and hat in one hand, and holding an open pair of surgical gloves in the other. There, on the counter, was the emesis basin that he'd be using to hold the treats. As soon as he saw me, his eyes brightened.

"Davis," he said happily, "you dressed up as a patient, just for me! That's so cool."

The nurse leaned over to me, quietly saying, "We didn't think you'd make it tonight."

"I wouldn't have missed it for the world," I said, as we went off down the hallway toward the first stop on our candy-begging expedition.

That whole doctor-as-patient experience taught me a great deal about what it's like on the other side of the stethoscope. Aside from the issue of adequate pain relief, I also experienced firsthand the ordeals of hospitalization, including the infamous pre-op bowel prep, medical student rounds, bed baths, the opened-back gowns, and narcotic-induced bowel and bladder dysfunction. I remember, for instance, not being considered for discharge home until I'd had a bowel movement after surgery. After about three days of stool softeners and laxatives, I remember sitting on the porcelain throne for two hours or more at a time until my legs and feet went numb, rocking back and forth, trying for my first movement. The mandatory bowel prep was also an experience to remember.

Along about bedtime, the nurse brought me some foul-tasting black stuff in a paper cup and said, "This is your Evac-Q-Kwik." Apparently, that is a brand name for the preoperative laxative that is given to clean out the patient's bowels before surgery.

I choked it down and said, "That was horrible."

The nurse just smiled that knowing smile and said, "Oh, you'll hate it, all right, but you haven't really got the whole experience yet." Then as she turned to leave, she added, "Tell me when it works."

About one in the morning, I had the sudden urge to use the restroom. I got up, went to the bathroom, and paged the nurse upon returning to my bed. "It worked," I told her over the speaker when she answered. About an hour later, the scene replayed itself. A sudden urge, a trip to the bathroom, just a little quicker this time, then back to bed. "It worked again," I said when she responded to my pressing of the button. Same thing forty-five minutes later when I informed her that it had done its magic once more. Then I settled into a pattern of running trips to the bathroom every thirty minutes or so, with more and more urgency each time. Liquid was all that I could produce by that time, and I was certain that I was "cleaned out," but the trips continued to be demanded by my now vacant bowels. I could hear the nurses laughing at the nurses' station each time I called.

Another experience that I remember from that surgery was, about the fourth day post-op, when I suddenly took chills and fever. My teeth were chattering, and I was shivering, lying there in bed. I asked the nurse for some Tylenol, and then some Motrin, hoping to decrease my fever before the nurse noticed it. I was certain that I was getting an infection that would prolong my hospital stay, and I didn't want things to go that way. After a while, I got fatigued and started to have some abdominal cramps (I hadn't had my first bowel movement yet.) When the nurse came in to take my temperature, I causally asked her how high it was. Much to my surprise, she just said, "It's normal." I waited for a while, and when the fever and chills started once again, I pushed the red nurses' call button and summoned the nurse. I asked her to take my temperature, and when she once again told me that I had no fever, I asked her, my teeth chattering, "What could be wrong with me if I have no fever?" She said, "Well, you've been on narcotics for over a week, between your pre-op time and your post-op time, and you haven't had any narcotics for more than a day now. I hadn't thought about it, but I hadn't requested any pain shots for a whole day. Of course! I was going through the symptoms of withdrawal. If that was what drugs feel like, I decided then and there that I would never misuse them.

On the second day post operation, I was awakened from my sleep by a nursing student. She was doing her clinical rotations and had been assigned to my post-op ward. I learned that it was her assignment to come and give me my first bed bath. I was unprepared for this experience and really didn't have much time to give thought to how I would react to the situation. She gathered a pan of warm water and a washcloth and began carefully cleaning my head ears and neck, as I lay in bed. She turned her attention to my torso; she left the sheets tucked in but lifted my gown without exposing my lower abdomen and keeping everything G-rated. She very carefully washed around my incision site, which was still very tender on my right flank. She then paused for a long time, swallowed a large gulp, and said, "I think I'm supposed to wash you all over." As I recall, I was heavily medicated and didn't even respond to her statement. As she lowered the sheets covering my lower half, I turned to her and innocently said, "Can we do this again when I feel better." Now in all honesty I only meant that her washing of my incision site had created some pain, and I really didn't want to continue the bed bath. The student however apparently misinterpreted my statement, threw the washcloth into the plastic tub, turned red, and ran out of the room. This was followed in a few moments by her clinical instructor, who came in demanding to know.

"What did you say to my student?" she asked me that at least twice, to which I fumbled with the answer.

All I really meant was that I would prefer to defer further irritation of my wound by this well-meaning student. Fortunately, my wife was present and witnessed this so that I was not in any trouble for excessive flirtation.

The other experience during this operation was during the pre-op phase, the night before surgery, when I was suffering through the gastrointestinal tract cleanout. The urology resident that was responsible for my care stopped by and said, "Do you mind if I have a med student examine you?" Of course, I replied that I didn't mind because I knew I was part of the educational process, being in a teaching hospital. This resulted in my experiencing no less than six consecutive rectal exams by various classmates who "just dropped by" because I was on the ward and available. I certainly learned what it means to be a part of a teaching program.

Have You Got a Longer Stick?

Training, as I did, in the Midwest had many advantages. The patients there provided a rich cross-section of personalities but were generally hardworking, dedicated to their families, and not inclined to complain very much about trivial matters. My experience at the VA medical clinic with an elderly farmer who was suffering from symptoms of gastric ulcer disease only served to reinforce this impression. The patient was in the outpatient clinic, the area of the hospital that served as a sort of a doctor's office where patients within the VA system could come to receive ongoing medical care. As a student, I served by examining patients, presenting my findings to an assigned attending physician, developing a treatment plan or a plan for further evaluation, and then explaining the findings and plan to the patient. I would then record the visit by documentation in the chart. With a concern about gastric ulcers, part of my planned evaluation involved sending the patient home with some small test cards, used for checking the patient's stool for unseen blood. The test, known as an occult blood test, required that the patient obtain samples of fresh stool and place a small quantity of the stool onto a specially treated paper test spot within a folding cardboard test card. The test card would then be returned at the patient's next visit, typically a few days hence, when a few drops of developer solution would be added that would result in a blue color showing up on the test spot if blood were present. Obtaining the specimens of fresh stool was always a critical but distasteful element of the patient's take-home instructions. I carefully explained my treatment and evaluation plan to the patient. I thoughtfully provided some latex rubber gloves and a few small wooden sticks intended to be used as a spatula to obtain the fresh stool from the toilet and to smear the sample onto the card surface. The sticks, about a quarter of an inch across and about five inches long, were standard issue and actually were provided by the test manufacturer for dispensing to the patient with their test cards. I gave the patient the cards, wooden sticks, and the instructions. The patient looked at the sticks thoughtfully, then raised his eyes to mine while reaching his hand out with the sticks, and said, "Have you got some bigger sticks?" Surprised by his reluctance, I thought to myself that he wasn't a very tough farmer if he was afraid to get his hands dirty by dealing with a little stool sample. I got up, reached into a drawer, and got some slightly longer and wider tongue blades, used to press the tongue out of the way during an exam of the oral cavity.

Handing him several, I said, "Here, these are a little bigger."

"Ya got anything bigger?" he asked.

Exasperated, I asked, "How big do you need?" His reply floored me.

"About yeh big," he said, holding his hands widely separated, indicating several feet in length. "Long enough for a one-holer." He laughed.

He was letting me know that, at his home, he didn't have indoor plumbing and would be obtaining the needed samples while using an outdoor toilet.

I laughed, as well, wondering out loud, "How do you plan on knowing which sample is yours?"

His reply was "I just thought I'd look down with a flashlight and pick the freshest-looking one!"

"No, you won't have to do that" was my comeback. I quickly made arrangements for the patient to take home some disposable bedpans, used in the hospital for patients who are too weak or debilitated to get up to use the restroom. He was actually very appreciative and took the supplies home to obtain his samples.

Cedar Rapids, Back Pain

One of the clinical rotations that I most looked forward to was my first rotation outside of the university-teaching setting. My schedule required me to arrange a rotation in family and community medicine with a primary care physician away from the medical school. I knew some physicians in rural areas but didn't want to travel very far due to my rotation falling in the winter and the unpredictability of the roads. I chose a physician that I knew that had a solo practice in a neighboring city. A variety of issues were considered in making this choice. The volume of his practice assured me a large exposure to a variety of clinical situations. The urban setting would allow me exposure to the specialty referral process away from the teaching hospital, and I knew and liked this physician. I had known him since my early teens and had even, at one time, had a brief none-too-serious courtship with his oldest daughter.

My goals for this rotation were several. Wanting to be a primary care physician in my future life, I hoped to see how family practice was successfully carried out. I hoped to see how a physician, outside of the university, carried on both a hospital practice and an office clinic. I knew all about making rounds on hospitalized patients but didn't know how a physician worked in an office setting, away from the central lab, radiology, and other supporting services. Within the hospital wards and clinics, the staff were all house staff, mostly future specialists. I had never really seen a family practice doctor, up close, since beginning my med school training. Oh, they existed at my campus but were all housed in a distant building and were rarely seen within the hospital halls. I anxiously wanted to have a family physician for a mentor. Finally, and most importantly, I had learned of the differences in types of complaints and problems that presented to office practices and hoped to see some of the more common and simple things that were cared for outside of the hospital setting. Was I cut out to be a family physician?

With that in mind, I made the drive the first day to the doctor's clinic. We had agreed to meet at his office at noon, and I'd spend the afternoon with him that day and make evening rounds with him at his hospital. We chatted about me, him, the practice, and my expectations for the time we'd spend together. His schedule was a bit pressing, and before too long, we had begun the afternoon's patient schedule. I'd followed him around for the first several patients, acting a bit like a lonesome puppy. I watched as he examined throats, measured blood pressures, examined skin spots, listened to lungs, and talked. He asked direct and pointed questions, seemed to arrive at a decision point, then, as he wrote out a prescription or checked off lab tests on an order sheet, he would talk to the patient. The patient, his family, the weather, the community, the illness, the planned treatment—all were potential topics of discussion. I liked this, my first experience in primary care as a member of the club. My first impression was very positive.

After several patients, seen at his side, I think he got a little bored with me following. He asked if I was ready to see a patient on my own. I jumped at the chance. Armed with my meager abilities as a diagnostician, but massive enthusiasm, he took me to an exam room and introduced me to the patient, making certain that the patient would be a willing guinea pig. My first primary care patient of "my own." I was to listen to the history, evaluate the complaint, arrive at a diagnosis, develop a plan, and return and report. He'd then check my work and help implement the treatment plan.

The patient was a male, late thirties, and a construction worker. His concern was for some back pain that had been bothering him for most of a week. Present over his lower back, he told me the pain was dull and achy but became sharper with movement. He had no leg weakness, and no numbness into his lower legs or feet. As I examined him, my mind was racing toward my differential diagnosis. I'd seen back pain at the university before. I knew the possibilities. My big university training was going to give me the answer and enable me to give great benefit to this, my first patient.

On exam, the patient indeed had lower back pain and tenderness. The tenderness was centralized over the mid and lower back and with pressure on the spine, he told me the pain was increased. He walked normally but had great trouble bending forward or sideways. No swelling or discoloration of the skin was visible. I finished my exam, gathered up my notes, and thanked the man as I headed out to the hallway and my waiting mentor. The physician was smiling broadly as we met outside the exam room door. Maybe he was looking forward to teaching me as much as I was looking forward to learning from him. Maybe he'd just heard a funny story from a staff member or pharmacy rep. Maybe he was just glad he'd gotten rid of me for a few minutes and had gotten some things done in my absence. Students can really slow you down, when you have one shadowing you. He was, nonetheless, smiling.

"What do you think?" was his first question to me. I relayed the results of my history. He declined to hear it all. I hadn't yet learned to tailor my history to only include pertinent positives and negatives, and he stopped me mid-ramble as I related the age of the patient's parents at their death as I started into recounting the patient's family medical history. Waving his hand in the universal signal to stop, he urged me on to the physical findings.

I communicated the areas of pain and tenderness, along with the absence of findings of significant nerve loss. I was thinking ahead, trying to include a couple of more possible additions to my differential diagnosis, the list of possible answers to the question, "What might the patient have, as an illness, to explain all the relevant historical and physical positive?"

I finally got to the point of the diagnosis, with his impatient urgings. My list began: osteoarthritis, septic arthritis, spinal tuberculosis, compression fracture of the spine, scoliosis, spondylolisthesis, and a list of about ten other esoteric diagnosis, most of which I had seen during my orthopedic rotation at the tertiary care university teaching center.

"*Hmm*" came his reply. He was, I thought, obviously impressed at my completeness in assessing and evaluating this, my first patient. I smiled. He smiled, then chuckled, and then laughed.

"Haven't you ever seen a back strain?" he asked. I flushed red.

No was my reply.

Midlaugh, he repeated "Spinal tuberculosis?—You've got to be kidding me!" then, "Let's get him some muscle relaxation and some physical therapy, so he can get back to work soon…Spinal tuberculosis?" He must have smiled at me three or four more times that morning, simply saying, "Spinal tuberculosis…"

I went on, day to day, learning an immense amount of medicine from that patient, caring physician. His had a busy practice and included inpatient hospital rounds, obstetrics, office surgery, and a busy office clinical practice. The most important thing that I learned, however, was the difference between medicine, as it was practiced "in the trenches," in a rural or community setting, as opposed to a teaching hospital. I learned to respect the adage that "common things are common, so when you hear hoofbeats, think of horses, not zebras." The idea being, horses are common while zebras are rare. He had a great influence on reinforcing my plans to enter the specialty of family medicine and to seek my postgraduate training—internship and residency—at a community teaching hospital, not a university center.

Unwrap the Suppository

At one point during my training as a medical student, I arranged a rotation in emergency medicine at a large urban hospital in a large midwestern city. The purpose of this rotation, which required that I travel four hundred miles from home and stay there for six weeks, was twofold. First, I would gain experience in a community hospital setting, and my wife, who was born and raised in that city, would have an opportunity for an extended visit with her family. Her childhood home was located just a few blocks from the hospital where I would be working, so we would be staying at her parents' home for the duration of the rotation. The emergency department wasn't particularly busy, but the relaxed patient flow gave me a lot of time to read up on each presentation of illness, to ask a lot of questions of the full-time staff, and to get a different flavor of medicine to compare to the high-risk and higher pressure of the university-teaching-center setting. Most of the patients who presented to the urban ED were run-of-the-mill ED patients who, in more modern times, would receive care in an urgent care center. They presented with the typical complaints: respiratory illness, work-related injury, after-hours and weekend injuries and illness, or they simply couldn't get in to see their primary care physician.

I wanted to maximize my experience, so I scheduled myself to be on duty six out of seven days. Thus, I found myself sitting at the ED front desk one Sunday afternoon, where I overheard a conversation between the admitting clerk and a waiting patient.

"How long until the doctor sees me?" was the patient's inquiry.

"She will be with you in about thirty minutes. She is with another patient, and she has one other patient to see before you" was the clerk's reply.

"She?…The doctor is a she?" the patient said rather excitedly.

"Yes, our doctor today is a resident physician from—" (naming one of the big teaching hospitals downtown) The patient was very keyed up, now, saying with a hurried urgency.

"Don't you have a male doctor or a male nurse that I could see?"

"No," the clerk replied, calmly.

"Our doctor today is Dr. M, who is a woman."

I could tell that the clerk had fielded this question before and actually seemed to be enjoying the discomfort and stress that her answers were causing the worried male patient. Then the clerk turned to me, tipped her head in my direction, and said, "Well, we *do* have a male medical student. I guess you could see him."

"Great!" said the patient, "I'll see him."

I thought to myself, *This is going to be interesting, I bet.*

A few minutes later, I picked up the chart and started toward the room, reviewing the patient's vital signs and reading the chief complaint from the top of the chart. The words were few and not very ominous, just a simple "talk to the doctor." Chief complaints are a very important part of the medical record. They are typically a written version of the patient's own words of why they came to be seen at that place and time. The patient's chief complaint helps the provider focus on what is important to the patient at that moment, what question they want answered, or what problem they want addressed at that visit. It is usually obtained from the patient as a response to some general question, such as, "What brings you in, today?" or "What can we help you with today?" It helps the provider direct attention to the patient's current problem in the most efficient way. This person wanted to talk, and he wanted to talk to a male.

Must be something very personal, I thought, as I opened the door.

"Hi, my name is Jim Davis, and I'm a fourth-year medical student working here today. How can I help you?" I said, in my most professional and cheerful voice. The patient was sitting on the exam bed, looking very apprehensive, but not pale, and no obvious blood or bandages.

"My thing," he began, "something's wrong, and it hurts." He was pointing at the zipper at the front of his pants.

I said, "What type of problem are you having exactly?" I continued.

He said, "You should just look. It's difficult to explain."

Oh great, I thought, *I'm going to see some big-city medicine—a sexually transmitted illness.* Quickly, I reviewed in my mind all the information I had learned about STIs, or as we called them back then, *venereal diseases.* I knew that the root word for *venereal* was the same as *venerate*—that is, Venus, the goddess of love. I was going to have to examine this guy for a sexually-transmitted disease. I began with some open-ended questions.

"When did you notice the problem?" I started. Over the next few minutes, I learned that the young man had noticed the onset of pain, some swelling, and irritation of the tip of his penis about three weeks earlier. He had discharge from the urethra, the opening at the very tip of the penis. He reported that sex had been painful, as had urination. The problem had worsened since it began, with some noticeable mild bleeding more recently. I dug into my memory for the appropriate questions regarding STI symptoms, in order to try to figure out which STI he had. I asked about the number of sexual partners he had. He replied that he only had one partner—his wife. He'd been married about a month. He had not had fever, chills, or any other noticeable symptoms. I handed him a gown and asked that he undress from the waist down, and I'd return for the exam. I gave him a few minutes to change, then reentered the room. He was sitting on the exam table and drew up the gown, exposing himself. The penis was a mess! The glans, the far end of the penis, was swollen, reddened, and had obvious drainage. I donned gloves for the exam and noticed that his undershorts had similar drainage evident in the front. With gloved hands, I examined him, checking for lymph gland enlargement, open sores, or other helpful evidence to aid me in the diagnosis. I was thinking of many things as I worked. Which of the STIs might this be? Would it be something that I'd seen before, in my limited experience, or would it be one of the rarer STIs found in larger cities? Where could I look up information that I'd need to make the diagnosis? What tests would be helpful? Finally, if it was an STI, what would his new spouse's response be to learning that her new husband had such an illness and had likely exposed her to it? As my mind actively pursued these questions and others, I looked closely at the glans. I noticed the raw skin had small linear marks that looked like abrasions or injuries to the glans. This appeared to be the source of the drainage, and the remainder of the penis—the shaft, the base, and the testicles were not involved. I did not see the typical lone ulceration characteristic of syphilis nor the localized urethral redness and drainage characteristic of gonorrhea and chlamydia. I was considering the possibility of the viral infection herpes simplex, which presents as a red-based rash, with draining blisters, and most closely resembled what I was seeing. Knowing that it was common for herpes to stay dormant in the nerves of the carrier only to come forth later as an eruption of painful and draining lesions, triggered when the nerves or skin surfaces are irritated. I wondered if one of the newlywed partnership had somehow reactivated a prior herpes infection that had resulted in the unusual lesions before me. I casually asked if the man's spouse had any similar symptoms. He replied that she had none. I asked further if she had any pain with sex or any discharge or other signs of infection.

This questioning awakened a memory in the patient, and he said, "Infection? Yeah, she had an infection, like at her exam before we got married, but she got it treated before we got married."

"Does she have any symptoms now?" I continued.

"No, she's completely cleared up" was his reply. I was a little disappointed because this information didn't fit with the diagnostic conclusion that I was moving toward, imagining how proud the resident physician would be when I presented this case to her, all neatly tied up with diagnosis and discharge plan, making her weekend shift all that much easier. Still, maybe I was onto something.

"Do you think she might still have some infection left over?" I asked.

"Well, you can ask her. She's out in the waiting room."

I discussed the situation with the nurse, who went to the waiting room to bring the spouse back to the exam area. After explaining my concerns about the possibility of infection spreading to her husband from an incompletely treated vaginal infection, she agreed to an evaluation and exam. Once again, I stepped out of the room while she changed into the gown for the exam. The nurse prepared her by explaining the proceedings and gathering the necessary equipment for the gynecologic pelvic exam. I came back into the room to find my new patient in her gown and her husband, who was now dressed, waiting in the room, with the wife seated on the exam table. The nurse assisted her into the position for the exam, lying supine with her feet in the metal brackets commonly called stirrups while I prepared the exam light, the equipment I'd need for obtaining cultures of any infection that I found, and readied the lubricant for the exam speculum. Once things were readied, I took my place at the foot of the bed, sitting on the rolling exam stool, explaining the procedure as I continued. Examining the external genitalia of the patient, I saw none of the typical clear blisters on a red rash that would indicate herpes simplex. I saw no evidence of a discharge from the vaginal entrance that would indicate chlamydia or gonorrhea, and I saw no evidence of the ulcer of a syphilitic chancre, the telltale lesion of syphilis. I gently inserted the speculum into the vaginal opening, pushing it back into the depths of the vaginal space. I pressed open the duck-bill-shaped jaws of the speculum to open the space and view the cervix, where infections were usually evident. As the jaws opened, I saw the problem, and the obvious solution. I leaned to my right, to make eye contact with the patient. She was apprehensively looking back at me.

"Did you have a vaginal infection that you treated before you got married?" I asked.

"Yes," she said, somewhat bashfully.

"Did you treat the infection with a vaginal suppository?" I asked, trying hard to keep my voice steady and professional.

Yes came the reply.

"Did you unwrap the suppositories before you placed them into the vagina?" I asked.

She leaned up, from her position lying on the bed, craning her neck forward as she with wide-eyed earnestness confirmed my suspicions. "Unwrap them? Nobody told me to unwrap them. They just told me not to take them by mouth."

The key to her husband's balanitis, the infection of the tip of his penis, was that she was placing vaginal suppositories into her vagina, complete with the aluminum foil wrapping that each one had wrapped around it. At body temperature, the suppository would melt, delivering the medicine that would treat her infection, but leaving behind the aluminum foil wrapper. Over the course of her treatment, multiple wrappers had been inserted and were still there, in the posterior pouch of her vaginal canal, just below the cervix. When she got married a few weeks previously and became intimate with her husband, the entry of the penis into the vagina compacted all of those wrappers into a little ball of aluminum foil. That little ball of aluminum foil brushed against the glans of her partner with every intimate thrust of a newlywed's sexual relationship. That led to the abrasions, scratches, and small lacerations that became infected. I removed the small wad of aluminum foil, treated the infected penis with topical antibiotics and a short period of abstinence, and reassured the couple that everything would be normal in a few days. I laughed myself silly as I related the elements of the case to the resident. Now, many, many years later, I still laugh to myself each time I relate the events of that case.

Fifty-Six-Hour Shift

In modern medical-training settings, controls are placed upon the workload of students, interns, and residents during their training. The limits are set upon the number of hours of consecutive work that may be required of those in training, as well as limits upon how many total hours per week may be expected from trainees. It was not always so, however, and medical schools and residencies have, in the past, been sites of long, continuous, and grueling hours of work in patient care areas. My longest stint of wakefulness came during a winter break when I was moonlighting by working in a clinical-laboratory setting within the university hospital. I was employed as a medical technologist in a laboratory and ran equipment that monitored the oxygen levels in the blood of babies who were being cared for in the newborn intensive care unit (NICU). As such, I would collect samples of blood from premature newborns and run it through a machine to determine the amount of dissolved oxygen or check on the levels of sodium, potassium, or chloride in their blood. These levels were critical to the proper care of these small infants. The laboratory was a satellite lab, located immediately adjacent to the NICU, and was staffed twenty-four hours a day and seven days a week to provide immediate results to the doctors working in the unit. I was scheduled for a twenty-four-hour shift, which was typical for the schedule at the time. Medical students were specifically hired to work as techs in that lab and were allowed to study or to sleep if not actually performing testing. It was usual to get some sleep during a shift. A cot was available that could be opened, barely fitting within the square footage of the cramped lab. Scrubs were typically worn, which served both as work clothing and pajamas. Every couple of hours, I'd be awakened to draw a few samples, run them, deliver the results, and then go back to sleep. A few kind residents would even go so far as to draw the samples for you, allowing you a few moments more of precious sleep. "No use both of us having to be up," they'd say. Occasionally, a baby would be having a bad time—crashing, as it was called, and serial testing would be required until the baby stabilized. Oxygen levels would be checked, the ventilator settings adjusted, and then a few minutes later, the test would be repeated. Sometimes it was an hour or two of steady work, followed by an hour or so of rest time. There was no TV available, so I usually got a lot of studying and textbook reading done during my shifts. It was pretty good work for a student. Besides learning to operate the laboratory equipment, blood drawing techniques could be learned, which were invaluable later when called upon to start difficult IV lines in infants and children. To this day, thirty years later, I still get asked to help start difficult IV lines on patients with small or invisible veins.

On this particular shift, a very premature infant was born who, due to the inadequate maturation of lung tissue, developed respiratory distress syndrome. This necessitated support of breathing by a ventilator and a special tube placed into the trachea, allowing a mixture of air enriched with oxygen to be pumped into the baby's lungs with each breath. The baby was unstable, which required constant readjustment of the ventilator followed by blood gas testing. This went on all day and into the night. The unit was particularly busy as well, with most of the thirty beds in the NICU holding newborns of various stages of prematurity and at various levels of critical care. After about twenty hours, I noticed that I'd been working steadily, with few breaks. Meals had consisted of a quick carton of juice or milk, and a quick half sandwich from the unit fridge in between test runs. I hadn't had any sleep at all for the whole shift. I wasn't worried, however, because it was the Christmas holidays, and school was not in session. I was not due on my new rotation until the first of the new year, and I'd be able to catch up on all my sleep. Anticipating some time to make some extra money, I'd sent my wife off to visit her parents for the holidays, planning to catch the after-Christmas sales for gifts, stretching our short funds even further. My children were very small at the time, and we'd decided that they wouldn't really know which day was Christmas, anyway, so they wouldn't notice that they'd be opening their gifts a few days later than everyone else. They'd still be able to play with gifts and share memories of the holidays despite their parents' disregard for the calendar.

Coming up on twenty-four hours of straight work, I thought about how I was looking forward to getting off duty and going home for some sleep. I knew that it was snowing outdoors. Reports were that the roads were getting slippery, and it was snowing ever heavier as time passed. I had planned to finish my shift, sleep a day to catch up, and then drive to the family holiday, refreshed and wealthier. Now I was beginning to worry about the drive.

With about a half hour of my shift left, my pager signaled for me to call the hospital operator. I thought my wife was calling to check on me and fill me in on the day's happenings. It was my replacement calling. He was at his parents' home, three hundred miles away, and unable to leave due to the storm, which was raging between us. It was not good news that it was still snowing three hundred miles away and outside the hospital and everywhere in between. He wasn't sure when he'd get out, and it was still an eight-hour drive for him to get through the snow back to the hospital to work. *Well, I'll just get a backup to cover his shift, but I'll continue to work in the meantime. More overtime…ca-ching,* I thought. Over the next few hours and in between running a series of lab tests, I tried calling each of the six other techs who worked in the lab with me. No one answered. This was, of course, before the era of cell phones, so the home number was the only option. No one had answering machines either. They weren't yet affordable enough for students. I checked with the lab supervisor. Not available, either. It was just me. I checked with other labs within the hospital, to see if there were any available techs with the proper training and found that most were short-staffed due to the storm and road closures. Even the emergency room was having difficulty getting patients in and out.

I hunkered down, resolved to make the best of the situation. I was increasingly tired, running on caffeine and adrenalin. Fortunately, the pace of requested tests did not let up, so I was constantly occupied with tests to run. The storm lasted about eighteen more hours, leaving snow drifts and piles several feet high. Snowstorms in the Midwest can leave the area paralyzed for hours to days. During one such storm in my youth, I recall that the governor of the state was surveying the snowfall results, traveling through the deep drifts of snow in an armored personnel carrier driven by a national guardsman. The governor's vehicle drove over a parked car, not visible under the deep snow drifts, and crushed it flat. Digging out from such a storm and opening the highways could take another day or so. Much of the remainder of that shift had become a blur, with my memory of the events somewhat clouded. I stoically continued to staff the lab, working with the NICU staff to care for those infants. I actually took on the challenge of seeing how long I could stay awake. The shift extended on through the second day. Forty-six hours, forty-seven hours, then forty-eight. I'd never been continuously awake for so long before or since. At fifty hours, I learned that my replacement had made it to a nearby town and was waiting for the road to open the last few miles so that he could drop off his family at his home and come to the hospital to relieve me. At fifty-two hours, he called from his home and was on his way. I remember finally lying down on the cot at that point, taking advantage of a short lull, and knowing that any testing that would be needed could be postponed until his arrival. The residents had become sympathetic to my plight and had lightened up the testing load by sending anything but *stat* testing to the central lab. The next thing I remember was standing on a bridge. I was on a bridge that crossed over the highway on the route by which I usually walked to my home from work. I became aware of the traffic, a long parade that was slowly snaking along on the plowed roadway on the highway below me. I was dressed only in short-sleeved scrubs. No coat. No gloves. It was very cold. I wondered how I had gotten there. I walked back to the hospital, to get my street clothes, winter coat, and house keys.

My replacement looked at me, amazed and asked, "Where did you go? When I got here, you woke up, greeted me, and then you walked out of here, kind of dazed, and said you were going home. I found your clothes here after you had gone."

I started home a second time, made it all the way this time, and slept for a day and a little more before making the four-hour drive to join my family for the holidays. Frankly, I was amazed at that feat, foolish as it was. I'd never been able to even come close to duplicating it, although I had, on occasion, gone more than thirty-six hours without sleep since then. Balancing shift work in the ED with family life sometimes required it, but it always resulted in a weeklong recovery cycle, during which I mostly felt like dog poop.

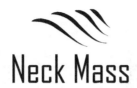

Neck Mass

During my fourth year, I had an experience in dermatology clinic that was noteworthy. In order to understand this, you had to understand that Iowa was predominately a farming state with very hearty people as its population base. Farmers' wives were notorious for being hard workers, dedicating themselves to the success of the farm. It was with that background that I walked into dermatology clinic to find my next patient who had a complaint of "neck mass." As I entered the room, I saw that she did indeed have a grapefruit-size mass from the left side of her neck. I was not experienced enough to really have a good differential diagnosis available but knew that this was a significant lesion and would likely require excision as a part of the treatment.

In the course of doing my evaluation, I was repeatedly struck by the size of the growth on the neck. It was fairly solid and had a substantial internal structure making it solidly attached. I couldn't get over the fact that this had not developed overnight, and so finally I said to her, "This looks like it's been present for a while. Why didn't you come and see me when it first started?"

Without missing a beat, she smiled at me and said, "You weren't born yet."

I chuckled at that but then asked the next logical question, "What made you finally decide to come into see the doctor?"

She said, "I was helping my husband plow the ground. I realized I couldn't turn my head side to side any longer to see if the plow was following me straight, so I told my husband, and he said, 'Well, you're no good to me here on the farm, then you might as well go to the doctor,'" and so, indeed she had done just that.

Late to Grand Rounds

During my rotation on urology, I had what was probably a never-to-be-repeated experience. Urology was a highly desirable residency at the University of Iowa due to the presence of the staff member who had invented the process for sperm banking. This contributed greatly to the eventual successful management of infertility from a variety of causes. While I busied my schedule with observation of a variety of surgical procedures, consisting mostly of holding the south end of a northbound retractor, it was also an opportunity to have other learning experiences and was my first introduction to organized grand rounds. The term *grand rounds* means "a gathering of physicians for the purpose of discussing a case from the near recent past where there had either been an adverse outcome, possibly death, or some other important teaching principle that each of the resident physician should understand thoroughly." We were invited as medical students to sit in on the grand rounds but usually not participate. Urology grand rounds were held on Sunday morning at about 8:00 a.m., so we as urology students tried to arrive at the hospital early, make our patient rounds, and be in our seats in the auditorium in time for the presentation of the case. A few minutes after grand rounds started during the middle of the first case being presented, there was a commotion at the side of the room, a resident was slowly coming in, finding a seat, and trying without gathering much attention to take his place in the crowd. The staff urologist stopped during midsentence, pointed in the direction of the resident, and said, "See me after grand rounds." There was a slight buzz that developed as we all contemplated what the residence's fate might be for being late and interrupting the process. I didn't actually overhear what became of that resident, however, there was a general memo sent to the full department, including all the medical students, which very tersely said, "Resident staff will no longer have intimate relations with their spouses on Sunday morning prior to grand rounds." What do you think happened?

La Crosse, OB/GYN

One of the rotations offered to seniors at the University of Iowa was off-campus rotation and OB/GYN in La Crosse, Wisconsin, at the Gundersen Clinic. I don't know if there were special requirements, but there was a selection process with the required application. I thought about this for a long time because I knew that I planned to have obstetrics be a part of my practice, and this additional concentrated experience was reported to be very beneficial to senior students going into the field of obstetrics for family medicine. This was balanced with the knowledge that it would require six weeks away from home, my wife, and children as well as driving back and forth to La Crosse.

I applied for the rotation and received notification that it had been awarded. La Crosse was located in the southwestern corner of Wisconsin along the Mississippi River in a very picturesque setting especially during the fall foliage change. The rotation consisted of six weeks of every-other-day schedule, which meant thirty-six on, twelve off, and moreover, every morning that you went to work, you would be staying that night on call. The result was an intense learning experience that promised lots of supervised deliveries as well as opportunities for learning surgical procedures. A couple of things were remarkable about the Gundersen Clinic, which was similar to the Mayo Clinic in nearby Rochester, Minnesota. One thing I remember was that on the OB floor, right outside of the elevator, was a six-foot-tall statue of a stork with a baby blanket in its bill, welcoming patients to the labor and delivery suite. The on-call quarters were located across the street in a separate dormitory area, but I don't really remember spending much time there because every free moment was spent either in the operating room, the delivery suite, or hovering in the emergency department looking for interesting cases.

I quickly settled into a routine of this schedule and started getting to know the staff. One of the staff gynecologists was Dr. M., the brother of a TV personality who was one of the stars of the show called *Route 66* and had equally dashing good looks. I started out on call for the delivery room, and my delivery count began to mount up. During the daytime, when not on call, I was obliged to review the surgery schedule and find interesting cases upon which to scrub. There were several procedures that I experienced for the first time in this environment. Time passed very quickly, and one day, I was scrubbed in the operating room with Dr. M. when I said something about my three children at home.

Behind a surgical mask, Dr. M. stopped, stared at me intently, and said, "You're married and have children?"

I replied, "Yes, three daughters."

The next thing he said surprised me as he asked, "Have you been home in the last four weeks?"

I replied that "No, I haven't visited home during this rotation."

And he very firmly told me, "It's Friday. Get out of here, go home, and visit your family."

As I recall, I didn't waste any time and certainly didn't have to be asked twice but made the six-hour drive back to Iowa City for a short visit to my family. I was back in the clinic on Monday morning and back on the labor and delivery and surgery rotation. It surprised me a bit to have been given this release from my duties, but I did enjoy the fall colors along the drive beside the river all the way to Iowa City. In all, it was a great learning experience with a lot of normal deliveries, interspersed C-sections, and new and interesting gynecological procedures.

One noteworthy encounter involved a young thirty-something wife of a lumberyard owner who was originally from Utah. She was a little uneasy during my initial evaluation for her impending delivery, which I initially attributed to reluctance to deal with a medical student. When asked about her apprehension, she averted her gaze, looking away, and said, "I'm afraid of what you'll think because I'm having my fourth child."

I said, "It's not up to me to judge how many children you have. I'm just here to make sure your delivery is successful and comfortable." She actually started to cry at that point because she had been so apprehensive about letting the medical staff know of the number of children she was having, feeling that they would be judgmental and in favor of much smaller families. I reassured her that she was not going to be subjected to such judgment at my hands, and I would do whatever I could to be sure that the nursing staff represented that viewpoint. She told me later that she had a very enjoyable delivery and thanked me for my nonjudgmental attitude.

Because the Gundersen Clinic was affiliated with a religious institution, elective abortions were prohibited, and I was therefore not required to participate in any of those procedures. I did however gather some experience with management of spontaneous miscarriage and the aftercare required by such patients. When the time came to travel back to Iowa City and return to my university studies, the fall weather was changing, and the curving roads along the Mississippi River were somewhat slippery for travel. I safely made it home having enjoyed the rich learning environment provided by this off-site experience.

Pimp

Internship is a time of intensive learning. As a medical student, you spend a lot of time filling in the huge gaps in your developing medical knowledge by watching others, mentors, go about the practice of medicine. Appropriately, the actual responsibility borne, in most situations, by a medical student is minimal. Medical students simply do not have the knowledge nor the experience to be primarily responsible for actual patient care decisions. Additionally, they lack the licensure, recognition by the state boards of medical examiners, to assume such primary responsibility. Once graduation occurs, however, the training method changes, and the new graduate, now called intern, often becomes the primary practitioner caring for the patients. Still with oversight by more experienced physicians, but much more intimately involved in the decision process and in the day-to-day care.

The intern's day usually begins with rounds—the process of visiting each patient on the service, accompanied by others on the team. The team consists of the interns, usually two or three, who share the responsibility for admitting and caring for patients, and one or more upper-level residents, and the staff attending physician—the practicing physician who is ultimately responsible for the patient. This means that the intern is the lowest-ranking member of the rounding team, which leads to an interesting process during rounds, wherein everybody but the intern can ask questions regarding some principle of medicine whether or not it relates to the care of the patient at hand in a process known as "pimping." Now I've known about pimping since medical school rounds, but I never knew the origin of the term. It turns out that it is an acronym for "put in my place" and refers to the low status of the intern (or student) pimped.

In a community teaching hospital, such as the one that I served my internship and residency, the teams may be smaller, containing fewer individuals compared to the teams of the larger university-associated teaching hospitals. In community hospitals, medical students are rarely present, and without them, the intern becomes, once again, the bottom rung of the team ladder. And, just as medical students experienced, they can become the object of relentless quizzing and questions during the time on teaching services. My internship was served at just such a community teaching facility. My first rotation as an intern there was surgery and was something that I had looked forward to eagerly. My prior experiences had taught me that I eventually wanted to be in a practice where I would be doing procedures of some sort. I did not want to be a surgeon, for a couple of reasons. One, because of the longtime commitments, selectivity, and condescending personalities of most surgeons that I'd met up to that point. I really didn't want to develop the personality of a surgeon.

Second, I really thought that I wanted more variety in my practice. I looked forward to having a practice that included a wide variety of patients and problems. Male, female, child, adult, and geriatric problems all looked interesting to me. I chose family practice because I knew that I could tailor my practice as I chose, to include all those demographic characteristics. I also wanted to deliver babies and take care of children. All my important medical role models to that point had reinforced that desire in me. My surgery team included another intern in my program, and two residents from the state university teaching hospital program in surgery. The residency, located about forty miles away at the university teaching hospital, sent their third- and fourth-year residents out to the community hospital, where they would be able to rapidly increase the numbers of surgeries that they were exposed to, away from the competition for cases at the teaching hospital. As a family practice intern, I wasn't interested in the more complex surgeries, such as bowel resections and mastectomies. I was more interested in hernia repairs, gallbladder removals, tonsillectomies, ear ventilation tube placements, and other less complex procedures that I might consider including among my own practice skills. It was a great trade-off. The other intern and I did all the easy cases, with no competition from the outside residents, and they did the more complex cases, with no competition from us. We worked as a team to provide the postoperative care, and we all rounded on the surgery service patients. The two interns, however, did all the admissions and the preoperative workups. The two of us were responsible for examining the patients on the evening before surgery (this was back before the advent of outpatient surgery, when patients still came in the night before a procedure and stayed a few to several days after the surgery). That rotation, a month in length, was highlighted by a reinforcement of my decision not to become a surgeon. While working with general surgeons in a community-hospital setting, I developed a new respect for the front lines of medicine. I learned that, away from the teaching atmosphere and competitive backstabbing of an academic training center, surgeons could be kind, caring, and competent professionals and great teachers—some, at least.

I do remember being on rounds with my team one morning and standing outside of a patient's room. This was a middle-aged female who had undergone a recent procedure and was rapidly improving in her postoperative care period. She had shown an abnormally elevated calcium level on her laboratory panel drawn that morning. She was not a patient that I had operated on, having had one of the university surgery residents in that capacity.

As we discussed her thus far smooth postoperative course, the most senior resident turned to me and asked, "Dr. Davis, what are the twenty-one causes of hypercalcemia?"

I thought quietly for a few moments, collecting my thoughts and going over in my mind the most common causes and coming up with about nine. He had caught me somewhat off guard. I had not anticipated that question because the patient was not really my own, nor had I known previous to that moment, about the elevated calcium level. My mind went back to my experiences on teaching rounds during medical school. How embarrassed students had been when presented with questions that they were unable to answer. I didn't want to relive any of those moments. In fact, I'd chosen a community teaching hospital just so that I would likely avoid those moments of embarrassment. Nine out of twenty-one, that wasn't even a passing score of 70 percent. I decided that the truth was the only way through this situation.

"I've only got nine causes coming to mind," I said, adding, "I'll have to go look up the others." After a minute or two of pursuing the question and laying on the discomfort a bit more, the two university residents began to laugh at each other.

The original questioner looked at me and said, "We only came up with six between us." I knew, at that point, that I would be able to successfully complete my residency. It was no longer about knowing everything; it was about knowing enough and knowing where to look for the rest. It soon became evident to me that medicine was not about books; it was about people and taking care of them.

Unidentified Jogger

Another interesting case for my internship-year rotation in the emergency department was a harbinger of things to come in the future in more ways than one. The first reason this case was preparatory to future experiences was because it forewarned of a career in emergency medicine the opportunity for which presented itself after six years. The second way in which it forewarned of my future professional experiences was that I learned that within the realm of emergency medicine, the ER physician will have many opportunities to solve mysteries regarding patients, mechanisms of injury, social circumstances, and many other kinds of situations presenting to the emergency department.

This case began in the ED of my training center when, at about dusk, the ambulance called and said they were transporting a young male patient who was the victim of an auto pedestrian accident that was also a hit-and-run. The patient was unconscious and had several visible injuries, and they gave an ETA of about two minutes. This case occurred during my internship year, but I had already experienced several shifts of coverage and, therefore, knew somewhat what I was doing, more or less. I did my initial patient survey with the attending present, and we quickly catalogued each of the visible or obvious injuries and began ordering the proper evaluations for those injuries, such as x-rays, CT scan, etc. The registration clerk was standing by the bedside awaiting the patient's name and other identifying information. The paramedics were not able to give any such information, and so the patient was simply listed as John Doe, and it would be up to me and the nursing staff to try to obtain further identifying information. The city police, investigating the accident, had no other information available on the patient and had no idea as to his identity. He'd been found along the side of the road, where he had apparently been hit by a car in the waning daylight and called in by a passerby as an unknown problem.

The patient appeared to be a young adult, late high school or early college age, and was clad only in a pair of running shorts, socks and running shoes, and a T-shirt. There was nothing descriptive about any of his clothing except the running shorts, which had the appearance of athletic shorts based on their cut and coloration. The colors used were those of one of the local high schools in the area with which I was familiar. The number was a two-digit number and appeared consistent with an athletic jersey number. There was no identification present on the person, and no other clothing was found at the scene. As I pondered how best to approach this problem of identification of this unknown victim, I also noticed a large scar on the anterior shoulder of the victim's right arm that had the appearance of a recent shoulder surgery procedure. Because the patient remained unconscious, I had little hope that I would find an easy solution to the patient's identification unless he woke up and began to talk to us.

As it turned out, this was just the first of many situations into which I was placed that required me to do further investigation into the real story of an emergency department patient. In most situations that one sees on television, the nurse or paramedic or EMT made certain statements at the time the patient appeared in the doorway to the emergency department that gave clues as to the patient's identity, history of events, and pertinent problem. This often was presented in a rapid-fire series of statements that tell us all the essential information needed in that situation, such as age, major problem, and complications. This was not the case however in the presentation of a real patient in a real emergency room, where, as in this case, none of that information was available.

In what essentially became a best-guess scenario. I telephoned one of my neighbors, who happened to work in the administration at the high school represented by this individual's running shorts. Fortunately, I found them at home and willing to help. I asked if he had a yearbook from the current year, which showed the high school football team, and he said that he did. He agreed to bring the yearbook over to the emergency department to review it with me. By the time the patient returned from x-ray and CT scan, I had the yearbook in hand open to the page displaying the football team and found the individual wearing the jersey number represented on the patient's running shorts. The individual in the photo had similar coloration of hair, and I used an ophthalmoscope lens to view a magnified image of the player's face. I determined that it could be a match.

Next, I looked at the medical record for a patient from within our hospital who had the same name and found that this patient had, indeed, undergone repair surgery for a shoulder dislocation the previous year. Bingo! Armed with this presumptive identification, I got the registration clerk busy on making calls to the patient's home and found that the patient was indeed out of the house, on a run to stay in shape. I took the phone from the clerk and told the mother, who answered the telephone, of the unusual nature of my call. I tried very hard not to raise alarm but suggested that she might want to come to the emergency department to help me confirm the identity of her injured son.

The patient later awakened, filled in some of the pieces of the story, and went on to a full recovery. This experience only served to show me a few of the challenges that lay in my future as a practicing emergency physician. It taught me to use my intuition, my skill as an examiner, the resources available to me in my neighborhood, as well as deductive reasoning on the order of Sherlock Holmes.

Do You Want a Pregnant Patient?

In a family practice residence, the residents in training are generally expected to develop a practice during their training. That is, in addition to providing care for hospitalized patients, who generally belong to other physician's practices and are admitted by those "attendings" into the hospital where the residents assist in providing the day-to-day care, residents are also expected to develop and maintain a practice of their own. This broadens their experiences and gives them more opportunity to develop decision-making skills as time passes. This is, of course, done under proper supervision by the residents' own teaching-physician attendings. Some types of patients, particularly obstetric patients, are in high demand for the residents. Such patients may originate in an emergency department encounter, whereby, if the patient says they have no current primary care physician and is in need of follow-up care from whatever problems happened to generate the ED visit, follow-up primary care may be arranged with the resident and would occur sometime afterward, in the medical offices of the resident. This accustoms the resident to the idea of an office-based practice and models the procedures that would occur in that setting.

One evening during my internship year, while on a shift in the emergency room at my teaching hospital, I was approached by one of the third-year residents with a proposition about seeing an interesting case. He was seeing a patient in the emergency department who had a complaint of foot pain and who happened to be pregnant, adding that she did not currently have a physician listed on the chart for her pregnancy and that if I would be willing to go provide care for her foot problem, there was a good chance that I could arrange to provide her prenatal care, as well. This third-year resident had developed a large model practice, already, including a large obstetric practice. In fact, it was well-known that he delivered more babies from his residency practice than did some of the practicing obstetricians from the community. I didn't want to look at his "gift" too critically, but I did wonder why he was being so benevolent, knowing as I did that, he generally accepted pregnant patients into his practice and that they were, in reality, quite sought-after. I picked up the patient's chart and went to take her history and perform her exam.

In her room, I found a woman in her late twenties, with an obviously pregnant tummy visible beneath her worn summer sleeveless dress. She was pleasant as I introduced myself. She looked just a little unkempt, but I passed that off as a product of the summer heat and that she likely belonged to a less-than-wealthy socioeconomic class. Neither problem served as a deterrent, and I was excited about the possibility of a new OB. She was sitting barefoot, legs dangling off at the end of the exam bed. She described her foot problem. She had been walking in flip-flop sandals for some time and had developed a blister on her heel, which had, she thought, become infected. I briefly reviewed her past history and her social history, learning that she was an unemployed single mom and that this was her third pregnancy. She had never married the father of her babies, and the same man had fathered all three. As I examined her foot, I noticed that she had moderate redness around a thin ulceration that was all that remained of the heel blister. The redness was just starting to spread upward along the back of the ankle, indicating a significant but not life-threatening problem. She would need some antibiotics and some soaking in warm water, which would soften the callous of her heel and increase the circulation into her foot. Also, she had some swelling of the foot, likely due to her pregnancy and the baby's head pressing upon the large blood vessels up in her lower abdomen, which had decreased the blood return from her legs, causing the swelling. Her blood pressure was good, and the baby had strong and rapid fetal heartbeat. I explained my treatment plan, asking her about medication allergies and current medications, with the answer of none to both lines of questioning. I then asked her who she was seeing for her prenatal care, figuring that, having already had two babies, she likely had an established care provider, and the third-year resident might have just been using that as bait to pass on the patient. To my satisfaction, she replied that she did not yet have a doctor for her pregnancy. I asked her about her pregnancy thus far, carefully probing for any signs of complications or abnormality that would place her at increased risk. Hearing none, I asked her if she would consider having me see her for prenatal visits, explaining that, as a family practice physician, I could conveniently provide care for her pregnancy and then for her and her child after the birth. She smiled and said that she thought that would be great.

Then her face becoming more serious, she said, "But I'm having twins, you know."

"Oh, I didn't know" came my reply, but in my mind, I thought over this new piece of information. *Wow, twins, a really rare find in a family practice experience. I can learn a lot from this patient and have the experience of delivering and caring for twins.* I couldn't believe my luck. Surely the third-year resident hadn't known this piece of information when he so readily passed over the patient. I was nearly gleeful when a thought suddenly occurred to me.

"If you haven't seen a doctor yet for this pregnancy, how do you know you're having twins?" I asked innocently.

"Oh" came her calm reply, "I can hear the two of them arguing in there…all the time."

"You can hear them…arguing…inside your abdomen?" I asked very tentatively, the realization of this woman's true problems hitting me like a wall.

"Yes," she said, "It's a boy and a girl, and they argue all the time."

The mother-to-be spent the next three weeks as an inpatient on the behavioral health unit, being medicated for her acute psychosis. During that time, her foot healed very rapidly, and her delusions and hallucinations cleared nearly as rapidly, and she continued to see me for her prenatal care after her discharge from the hospital. She remained stable throughout her pregnancy and delivered a healthy baby girl, which the state's department of family services promptly removed from her care, placing the baby with foster parents, as they had her previous two children. Last I heard from her, she was still working on keeping on her medications so that she could try to get her children back.

Moonlighting

The process known as moonlighting may or may not be offered to residents during their second and third year. At many residencies, moonlighting is considered a way of increasing exposure to patient care and is deemed to allow a broader experience while still under control of the residency. At other institutions, it is a totally independent function and is done independent of the residency and oftentimes without their direct knowledge. In the third case, moonlighting may be considered inappropriate due to the excessive workhours placed on the individual. At my residency, it was supported and encouraged. We had two moonlighting sites set up one in Logan, Utah, and the other in Burley, Idaho. Only second-year residents were scheduled in Logan, and only third-year residents were scheduled in Burley. In order to work at either location, one first had to pass their national board exam and become formally licensed within the state of practice. This meant that, as a resident, I had licenses issued by the states of Iowa, Idaho, and Utah.

In addition to supplementing our patient care experiences and learning how to obtain consultation and referral for follow-up care, there was always the extra income, which was beneficial to a young physician just starting out in practice especially with the family. This allowed my wife to spend time with our children rather than taking a job outside the home.

At the time, both moonlighting sites were similar consisting of rural-practice settings without full-time emergency medicine practitioners, with the care being provided by family doctors, who typically took call during their office hours and responded directly to the emergency department when an emergency presented to the hospital. Coverage by a moonlighting resident would typically start on

Friday night at a designated time and continue forty-eight hours until Sunday night at the same time, when the practice would revert back to the local physicians. The visiting residents would stay in the hospital for that forty-eight-hour block and be available for evaluation and treatment of any patient presenting to the emergency department. Occasionally, other single sites would be offered to third-year residents on an individual basis, which might include making rounds on Saturday and Sunday on hospitalized patients. Several of these moonlighting opportunities led to full-time practice positions being offered to the residents upon completion of the residency training.

A couple of experiences show there was not always "all work and no play," however, as evidenced by the recollection I have of sending a member of the nursing staff one Saturday evening, when we weren't otherwise busy, on an errand to purchase ice cream and toppings to make sundaes as a treat for the staff. The plan was that we collect money from everyone, send a nursing student to the local Albertsons store to purchase the supplies, and upon her return, we would create the treats in emesis basins to eliminate the need for dirty dishes. I recall that it was winter time and that she was wearing a green coat as she left the emergency department.

Immediately after she left, several of the group got together and made plans to play a joke on her. I called the local Albertsons and asked to speak to the manager. When he came on the line, I told him that there was a young lady in a green coat in the ice cream freezer section whom I had seen stuffing items into her pockets with the obvious intent on leaving without paying for them. He very firmly said that he would look into the situation and check for that individual. Having baited the trap, we all stood by waiting for the return of the unsuspecting student. After several more minutes of patient waiting, she arrived back at the emergency department, shopping bags in hand with all the needed supplies. When asked how things went at Albertsons, she replied that she had changed her mind and had gone instead to Safeway and found her shopping uneventful. We enjoyed the ice cream but not as much as we would have enjoyed it had she been stopped by the store manager.

This good-natured joking was not always instigated by me however. On one occasion, I came to work the shift at Logan on a busy Friday evening. There was a constant flow of one patient after another in what seemed to be a never-ending line up at the front desk. I had driven from my residency to Logan and had immediately proceeded to see the first patient, who was already waiting, without taking a rest stop, which was not all that unusual. It was a couple of hours before I even had an opportunity to take a break, and by that time, my bladder was screaming that it needed some attention. There was a small restroom attached to the room that was used for the residents' overnight stay, and I walked into that room without even turning the lights on because I was in such a hurry to empty my bladder. In the dark room, I did not see the trap that the nurses had set for me. They had covered the seat of the toilet with tightly stretched saran wrap so that when I sat down unaware of the invisible plastic layer and began to empty my bladder, I was surprised to find urine flowing everywhere. This unregulated bladder relief was accompanied by the inability to stop the stream once started. We all had a good laugh, at my expense, and I immediately had to change into green scrubs. This was only the first of a long series of practical jokes between the resident physicians and the nursing staff.

Nurses

One of the reasons for selecting the particular residency that I chose was because it offered the opportunity to learn some surgical procedures that I had interest in providing to my patients and it was located within a healthy population that had a high rate of pregnancy and delivery so that I could also learn more about obstetrics. I'd mentioned before that I was planning on doing obstetrics in my practice, and so I selected a residency that while my classmates, back at Iowa, were getting to deliver twenty-five or thirty babies during the entirety of their residency, I was, through my residency experience, able to do many times more than that. In fact, during one month of my residency, the teaching hospital where I was working experienced a record number of births due to the scheduling of the annual meeting of NACOG (National Association of Obstetricians and Gynecologists) on one of the islands in Hawaii, which meant that all the OB/GYNs had planned on closing down their practice and most of them leaving town for the duration of the meeting. This meant that the labor and delivery service was very, very busy and that I had a record-breaking experience.

My first night on call, however, I learned a valuable lesson that I did not soon forget. I really couldn't recall the details or what I did to create the problem, but I remember the problem started just after midnight when I had delivered a baby, written my note, tucked in the patient, and went to the on-call room to catch a little sleep. I never really did hear the details of my exact transgression, but I became aware of a problem about thirty minutes later, just as I was falling asleep, with the ringing of the phone. The phone call was from the labor nurse who was caring for the patient that I just delivered. She was calling to tell me that the patient was stable and her bleeding was controlled. The patient was not having much pain, and the baby had been out with the mom and had successfully nursed. I thought this was great information to have, very reassuring, and I thanked the nurse and proceeded back to try to get some sleep. About thirty minutes later, my phone rang again. I was being telephoned by the same nurse, who gave me essentially the same report. A stable patient, in no pain, no significant bleeding, in fact, she said the mother was sleeping well. I still didn't catch on, thinking that it was just good manners or good nursing care or both to keep me so well-informed.

It was at the receipt of the third and fourth phone calls that I put the pieces together and realized that this nurse was attempting to teach me a lesson by continually interrupting my sleep with phone calls that, while reassuring, were probably unnecessary. After the fourth or fifth phone call, I asked, "Is there something wrong? Did I do something to irritate you?"

It was then that she relented, saying, "Yes, you did." Either she didn't ever tell me exactly what I did, or I'd forgotten it, but I'd never forgotten the lesson about the power of the nursing staff, especially when it came to interrupting your sleep. The value of this lesson became more fully apparent during my years in emergency medicine when I discovered that nurses could literally make or break your career by keeping you from discharging a patient who wasn't ready for discharge or probably shouldn't be discharged because of the complication. However, since that early experience with a labor and delivery nurse, I tried to make sure that nurses were always kept on my good side. I found, over the years, that nurses responded well to bribes and treats but most especially to sincere respect. Considering them to be part of the team, seeking their input and opinion, and listening to what they say had kept me out of a lot of trouble over the years. Looking back, I had that delivery room nurse to thank for that valuable lesson.

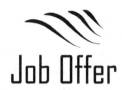

Job Offer

As I neared the end of my training program, I had identified the community where I planned to open my first practice, in partnership with another family physician who had first opened his own practice a few years earlier. He had rapidly grown very busy and found that he needed to take on a partner. I first met this physician when I was on a month-long newborn-intensive-care-unit rotation and was on call for the newborn transport team, a group consisting of a transport nurse, neonatologist (a specialist in newborn care), the resident currently on the service, and an ambulance crew who drove the ambulance carrying the equipment and other team members to some remote site to pick up premature or otherwise ill newborns, bringing them back to the teaching hospital for specialized care. In more modern times, the actual transportation is most often provided by a helicopter that is specially equipped for the purpose, but in the late seventies, standard ground ambulances were more common.

Twins had been delivered prematurely at a hospital located about fifty miles distant from the teaching center. They were doing well, but their incomplete development meant that they needed close observation and supplemental oxygen for their underdeveloped lungs, at least, for as long as it took them to mature. At the remote hospital, I first met my future partner, who had delivered the twins. I was impressed by his ability to provide excellent stabilizing care for the preemies and to keep them healthy until the arrival of the transport team. I learned later that he was similarly impressed with my care and my concern for the newborns, as well as my bedside manner with the babies' mother and father. He also appreciated my manner with the local staff, avoiding the "ivory tower" arrogance that sometimes accompanied such a transfer—the transfer team seemingly swooping in to "save the day" and leaving the local providers feeling somewhat behind the times or incapable of providing good care. Regardless, about a week later, I received a phone call from the transferring physician, which I thought simply meant that he was checking on the progress of the twins, who were essentially nearly ready for transfer back home with the parents. Actually, he said, he was calling to ask me if I had yet selected a site for my future practice. In fact, I had been considering going into practice right there, in the community where the teaching hospital was situated. I had been invited to join the practice of some former residents, graduates of a year previous, who already had a busy practice, and needed to add another provider. I had always thought I might want to practice in a smaller community, but this ready-made practice, with partners that I knew, from a training program that I knew, seemed up to that point, ideal. I told him of my tenuous plans, telling him that I hadn't really made any firm agreement yet, but that it was under consideration. He was a good salesman, telling me of the great benefits of small-town practice and life in a small, safe, and friendly community. I agreed over the phone to discuss the offer with my wife and to call to set up a dinner, where I could meet other physicians in the community and further discuss his offer. So I found myself, in my last few months of my residency, with a firm agreement in place to begin practice in a small community in northern Utah and, aided by the small town hospital administrator, with an opportunity to sell my house near the teaching hospital and purchase a house in what was to become my new community. It would mean commuting back to the residency site each day, a round trip of about a hundred miles or so, except on nights when I was on call, about every third night during my third year, when I would just sleep overnight at the teaching hospital in the on-call quarters shared by the residents. Normally, as a third-year, I would be able to take call from my home, by telephone, but I would need to be within fifteen minutes of the teaching hospital to take the call, so I would sleep there rather than at home.

Bee in the Back Seat

One night, I was on my way back home, after two busy days, interrupted by a busy night on call. It was late spring, and the weather was warming. I was on the last leg of my commute, having just left the interstate and driving along a five- or six-mile straight road leading to my new community. I was cruising along the empty highway, windows down, radio up, happy to be getting home at last. Suddenly, a huge bee flew in my window, brushing across my neck as it entered the rear of my car. I could hear it buzzing in the back but couldn't see it despite repeatedly checking my rearview mirror. It was close, over my right shoulder, but I couldn't visually see it. Finally, I glanced over my right shoulder to try to locate the insect. Inadvertently, in looking to the right, my hands turned the steering wheel slightly to the left, causing my vehicle to cross the center striped line. Fortunately for me, the highway was completely vacant except for one car, which had enough distance to react to my error and slow and pull over to the shoulder, raising a dust cloud, but allowing me to easily and safely pass by. Unfortunately, the car had red lights atop it and was driven by a highway patrolman. After recovering, I immediately pulled to the side of the road, slowed, and stopped. I watched as the patrolman wheeled a U-turn, turned on his overheads, and pulled in behind my stopped vehicle. He got out and approached my driver's side door. I had opened my door and was in the process of getting out to avoid further contact with the bee buzzing around in my car's back seat. Adrenalin pumping and in his most forceful law officer voice, he demanded to know why I had forced him off the road, asking the rhetorical question of whether or not I was trying to kill us both. Paled by my own adrenalin response, I turned to my opened door and pointed to the seat, saying the single word, "Bee!"

He stepped forward, hand on his weapon, saying in a still loud and excited voice, "Bee? What bee?"

Just then, as if guided by some unseen comedy-show director, a huge bumblebee lumbered out of the opened door, hovering a foot or so off the ground, buzzed around the officer's legs, and then off into some roadside field. The close proximity of a bee so large caused the officer to do a sort of a dance, lifting one leg, and then the other, in an effort not to be stung.

Turning to me, he said, "Well, I've got to give you a ticket, but under the circumstances, I'll make it a warning ticket."

Later, in my subsequent years in the community, I got to know that officer very well. His wife came to work as a receptionist in our office. He was a regular patient, and we worked together to provide care for many of the local residents when they were injured in traffic-related incidents. A couple of years later, he was retelling that story of our first meeting, and I told him, jokingly, of course, that I always carried a jar in my car, with a huge bee in it, and if I was ever pulled over for a traffic stop by an officer, I simply unscrew the lid, releasing the bee into the car.

"It works every time," I said. "I never get a ticket."

Infant Gastrointestinal Bleed

As part of my training program, I was encouraged to gain additional experience in the practice of medicine by providing weekend coverage to emergency rooms. This was recognized and promoted by my residency as a learning experience. Typically, it involved traveling some distance to a smaller, rural emergency department and providing coverage for all or part of the weekend. While I was expected to provide general coverage, I also had backup coverage from all the physicians in the community. During one of these occasions, a patient presented was a newborn who was reported vomiting blood.

I entered the room to take the history from the mother and to examine the child. I found a mother holding an infant in her arms. The child appeared healthy, pink, and vigorous. I asked the mother about the reported vomiting. According to the mother's history, the child had vomited several times in the past two or three days. Each time, the vomitus was pink with blood. There was no history of vomiting without the mother seeing blood. There was no history of dark-black stools, a finding that would have indicated that the blood had been mixed with stomach acid and digested while passing through the baby's intestine. I asked about the mother's pregnancy and delivery, both of which were uneventful. The baby had stayed in the hospital the usual time period and had been released healthy with the mother. The course at home had been uneventful, as well. The infant had had no illness, was taking no medications, had been examined during the normal newborn exams, and there were no reported abnormalities. For all purposes, this was an apparently normal infant. I asked about food intake. The child had been growing normally, with normal intake. The mother was nursing the child at regular intervals. The baby seemed to eat vigorously, to become full, and did not always vomit after feedings. Sometimes, however, after eating, the child would cry, seem to have colic, drawing her knees upward, and then vomit the recent feeding, tainted with blood. The mother had no breast soreness and no sores on the nipples.

Pink or bright-red bleeding that accompanies vomiting can occur from ulcers in the stomach, if the vomiting occurs immediately after eating, as in this case. Otherwise, if the blood sits in the stomach for very long, it turns dark, appearing black after mixing with the stomach acid. It can take on the appearance of coffee grounds. Another place that bleeding can occur is in the lower esophagus, the hollow tube that carries the food from the mouth to the stomach and contains a muscular valve that keeps the food in the stomach. Sometimes a small tear can occur in the lower esophagus if the child has an area of irritation or blood vessels that are abnormally prominent. In the latter case, the blood vessels can erode and bleed. Or newborns can be born with a developmental defect in which small- or medium-size arteries can be directly connected to corresponding veins, resulting in veins, which are normally low-pressure vessels, bulging and prominent from higher-than-normal pressure provided by the arteries. This is called an AV malformation and is somewhat a rare condition. In any of these cases, the bleeding can be very brisk and result in dangerous blood loss very rapidly. This baby, however, looked quite the opposite. While we were talking, the mother asked if she could feed the baby. I was anxious to solve the source of the bleeding, so she nursed the infant while we continued to talk. After several minutes of nursing, the child seemed fine, and the mother switched sides, feeding from the other breast. I was really wondering what could be causing this unusual situation when the child suddenly pulled away from the breast, turned very pale, and vomited pink milk all over herself and her mother. I was amazed. I left the room to call the regional children's hospital. I knew that the child needed a procedure for looking into the esophagus and stomach to determine the source of the blood. I knew that the small community hospital was unlikely to have a scope that would be small enough to fit in the gastrointestinal system of this small of an infant. I telephoned the children's hospital and spoke to the emergency department. Given the significance of the blood loss and the grave possibilities of rapid bleeding, the receiving hospital wanted to send a helicopter with a flight team for the transfer. I agreed with the transfer and proceeded to finalize the arrangements. Because of the distance of the transfer, I felt that the baby should forgo any further feeding to reduce the possibilities of more vomiting while in flight. Any vomiting in the small enclosed spaces of the helicopter could result in compromise of the infant's airway or other complications. The mother, of course, wanted to travel with the infant, but that would not be possible on the helicopter flight. She would need to be temporarily separated from her child for the duration of the flight, about ninety minutes. The mother, meanwhile, would drive to the hospital with her husband. It would be some time before she would arrive at the hospital, and I suggested that we send some of her breast milk along with the flight crew, to feed the baby after arrival at the receiving hospital. I arranged for a breast pump from the labor and delivery department, so the mother could gather her milk to send along. I left the mother and patient alone while I finished the paperwork for the transport. When I returned to the room, the mother had collected the breast milk and handed me the bottle. The milk was pink. I suggested a careful exam of the breast and found absolutely nothing abnormal about the breast or nipple. When the mother manually expressed milk, however, normal milk was produced from the left breast and normal milk was produced from the right from all the tiny ducts of the nipple, except one—it produced blood. It was the mother who had a small hemangioma, an abnormal collection of enlarged capillaries, a short distance inside the nipple. Every time the child would suckle, the hemangioma would release blood into the baby's digestive tract, mixed with the milk. The other breast, being normal, provided normal milk. Thus, the child would only vomit after being fed from the right breast. I canceled the helicopter. Another difficult case solved.

Primary Children's Medical Center Code Blue

While working at a specialty children's hospital during my internship, I was assigned to be the on-call house officer every third night and had to be available, at the hospital, for a twenty-four-hour period. At this time, I was the most-junior physician in the hospital and ended up with all the *scut work*, such as drawing blood, looking at lab results, chest x-rays, interviewing new admissions, and so forth. This placed me in close and frequent contact with all the nursing staff. In the process of providing care to very ill children, it was easy to develop a camaraderie, and that sometimes led to teasing and joke-playing. After a six-week rotation, I knew all the night nurses, and they knew me. I had played my share of tricks on them, and they were ready for paybacks.

It was my last night on call, a quiet night, and I was catching up on my charts before changing to another assignment at the end of the following day. Suddenly, my concentration was broken by my pager's tone telling me of an incoming message. To my horror, I heard those dreaded words *code blue, intensive care unit*, followed by the message being repeated twice more. I ran down the hall and up the two flights of stairs. Elevators were always too slow. I arrived, breathless, at the doorway of the ICU. I saw the nurses hovering over a small, pale body, lying still and lifeless on the warming bed. One nurse was hanging an IV line. Another was gathering medications, and a third and fourth nurse were doing CPR on the baby's chest, compressing the chest wall with her index and middle fingers to provide blood circulation in the absence of the baby's own heartbeat and using an inflatable bag to provide artificial breaths to the baby's mouth by way of a tight-fitting mask. I asked about the history. They told me that the baby had been admitted a day earlier, to another team's service, with the diagnosis of congenital heart disease. I asked about what had been done so far and how far into the ACLS procedures they had gotten by that time. The charge nurse informed me that they had good ventilations, could hear good breath sounds, and that the chest was rising with each breath. I quickly checked the electronic monitor and asked the nurse providing the chest compressions to stop for a moment, so I could determine the baby's heart rhythm. She stopped, and I saw that the monitor was showing a steady flat line moving across the screen. I immediately recalled the standard procedure for resuscitation of a pulseless infant. Suddenly, I noticed that the baby was really rather pink for a dying infant. I reached over to pinch the skin, to see if the blood was circulating through the extremities. I noticed, to my chagrin, that the "baby" was plastic. They were busily performing CPR and resuscitation on a manikin that is used for educational purposes, commonly named Resusci Baby. The nurses collapsed into fits of laughter. I was flushed with embarrassment. I'd been had. What goes around, comes around.

Burley, ER Blood Draw

When working in the emergency department, an ED physician is usually in the position to be of assistance to law enforcement officers. On rare occasions, however, the ED physician can find him or herself acting as a patient advocate first, and this can land the physician in opposition with law enforcement.

On a weekend moonlighting shift in Burley, a city some distance from my training center, I was working through the usual Saturday night's steady flow of patients. Around 11:00 p.m., a police officer appeared at admitting with a young man in tow. The officer wanted the patient checked into the emergency department to get a sample of blood drawn in order to determine the level of alcohol in the patient's blood. Allegedly, the youth was celebrating his twenty-first birthday a few hours early, had gained entry into a bar, had been drinking, and then was apprehended while driving his car from one bar to another. He was suspected of both underage possession/ ingestion of alcohol and operating a motor vehicle while intoxicated. He would turn twenty-one at midnight, one hour hence. The problem was that the youth did not want his blood drawn, of course, and was refusing to have the lab poke him for the blood draw. The officer then requested that, as the attending physician, I draw his blood and submit the sample for analysis for a legal blood alcohol level. I spoke to the young man alone in the room without the officer and confirmed his unwillingness to have me draw his blood. This set up a peculiar situation.

According to the laws of the state where I was working, I could not properly render care to a minor child without the permission of that child's parents, and this was a policy that I tended to follow, unless there was a threat to the child's life or limb. Also, in that state, under the principle of implied consent, whereby when an individual assumes the position as a driver of a motor vehicle, they imply consent to be tested for the presence of alcohol, and no further consent is required. Officers can obtain that information, usually by a breathalyzer test, without the driver's permission and not violate any search and seizure rulings. The lad told me that his father was an attorney and would sue me or have me charged with assault if I drew his blood without his (the father's) permission. This was obviously a ploy because, although the young patient was clear thinking and witty with regards to his legal defense of the DUI, he also had a strong odor of alcohol and appeared intoxicated to my experienced eyes. I suggested a compromise with the officer. In about fifty minutes, the patient would be of legal age, and I would no longer be required to have the permission of his parents, and I would then draw his blood for the lab test. The officer replied with his concerns about the possibility of the blood alcohol dropping over the passing time because the patient would continuously metabolize the alcohol during that time and the end result might be a lower or even normal blood alcohol level. He was, therefore, anxious to have the blood drawn immediately, so as to document the alcohol level at its highest point. I explained my position, and he explained his.

His position, as he stated it was "Either you draw this patient's blood now, or I will arrest you for obstruction of justice and failure to comply with the order of a police officer."

I told him that I didn't think he would be well received by the community if he removed the only emergency physician from the only hospital in the community on a busy Saturday evening.

We were thinking over each other's positions when the receptionist came back to me and said, "There is someone having trouble in the parking lot. They don't seem to be able to park their car."

She had been watching on the closed-circuit security camera as a driver of a sedan had repeatedly tried to park their car in a small parking space. The driver would head into the slot, a little misaligned, then stop, and back up, straighten the car a little, then try again. I thought it might be an elderly person who had difficulty seeing. Normally, I would let one of the other staffers go check out the situation and assist, but I wanted and needed a little space from the police officer who was standing at the desk at the moment, so I said I'd go out and help.

I approached the car from the passenger side and noticed, to my surprise, that it wasn't an elderly person, but a young woman, in her late twenties at the wheel, with a man, about her same age, in the passenger seat, leaning over on her shoulder. His presence against her shoulder was impairing her ability to turn the steering wheel enough to fit the car into the parking spot. I rapped on the window and opened the passenger side door.

"Do you need some help?" I asked.

Rather calmly for the circumstances, she pointed at her passenger and said, "He's been shot."

The nurse, who had followed me outside, also in need of some fresh air, ran back to get a bed and some help. I donned some rubber gloves and lifted the man out of the car seat and onto the arriving portable bed. He was breathing, barely. He was making some groaning noises. I didn't know where the gunshot had entered his body but looked him over for obvious blood as we reentered the ED on a full run. The overhead page for a trauma team activation brought all kinds of help, including respiratory therapy, lab, x-ray, and another physician who happened to be making late rounds on a patient. I immediately found the gunshot entry point on the right side of the patient's neck, just above his collarbone. I stabilized his neck with a protective collar as the nurse started an IV line in his arm. I rapidly sedated him and placed a tube in his airway to keep it open so that we could assist his breathing. X-rays showed his spine and trachea to be normal and showed a small caliber bullet still lodged in the soft tissues of his neck. Thus stabilized, I completed the exam of the rest of his body and began to resuscitate him with additional blood and fluids. When I had finally turned him over to the surgeon on call, I returned to the front desk. It was after midnight.

"Where's the cop and the DUI kid?" I asked. No one knew. I never did hear how he handled the situation with the attorney/father, but he didn't take me off to jail, so I was happy.

"Wolf" Up the Canyon

Part of residency training is learning to work with different personalities among the staff attending physicians. At my training hospital emergency department, the staff was very good, in general, but because the specialty of emergency medicine was still fairly new, all these physicians had come from prior practice settings into the area of emergency medicine.

One such emergency specialist was by original training, a thoracic surgeon. Now that begs the question as to why a thoracic surgeon, if successful in that subspecialty area, would practice emergency medicine. I arrived at the conclusion that either he was burned out from the years of practicing in the ER, or that he wasn't very successful in the practice of thoracic surgery and made his way into emergency medicine by default.

Now it's important to say that, currently, most emergency department physicians are very capable and have chosen that as the primary specialty, but in the early days of emergency medicine, this is not necessarily the case. Many people became ER doctors through a different route. I myself, as you can see, started in the area of family medicine but saw the importance of emergency medicine as a specialty, and so early on, I took my board certification in ER and began practicing that specialty exclusively.

Another physician in question was actually a very good emergency physician; he just had no people skills to speak of. In fact, he was a bit of an "odd duck." One example of this was that he would ask random questions out of the clear blue sky that were totally unrelated to the topic at hand such as asking me one evening.

"Jim, did you know that during World War II, the Japanese sent hot-air balloons to the United States, and one landed outside of Tremonton?"

I was not sure where his head was before, during, or after that comment, or why he chose that moment to ask that random question.

Anyway, I was on duty in the ER in the community of Ogden and was seeing patients as they presented to that level II teaching hospital emergency department. I picked up a chart, read the chief complaint, and found that the patient was complaining of abrasions, lacerations, and was a survivor of an attempted assault. As I was taking the history of this young woman, I learned that she had found herself in a compromising situation while on a date and had run away from the perpetrator while at a romantic parking site somewhere up Ogden Canyon. She gave the name of the restaurant with which I was familiar, as the site of the assault. I was familiar with its reputation as an after-hours parking site for the local younger crowd. The patient turned out to be a young woman in her early twenties with some abrasions and smudges on her face and appeared a bit disheveled.

I cheerfully asked her, "How can I help you?"

She said that she had been parked near the restaurant in a dark and secluded area when she felt that things were getting out of hand physically with her date, and she fled the vehicle into the parking lot and across the parking lot into the adjacent brush.

In the process of finding her way through the brush, she had suffered the abrasions and scrapes but had managed to get free and flagged down a passing motorist, who brought her to the ER. She had not been physically assaulted otherwise but had suffered multiple small barbed stickers from some of the bushes, and these were liberally present in the clothing of her lower extremities and arms. I checked her generally for other major injuries and found none, so I asked her how I could best help her. She desired to have the remnants of the cockleburs removed, and I agreed that she should have that done before they became inflamed, infected, or both.

She appeared to have literally hundreds of small splintered and woody cockleburs on the skin of her legs and arms. I obtained some magnification and some cleaning solution and set about to the task of removing the, literally hundreds, of attached foreign bodies. She was wearing summer shorts, so this was easily accomplished without having to make her disrobe. I was happy for this because I felt, due to her near escape from the recent assailant, she probably had been through enough emotional turmoil for one night. With the help of a bright spotlight and a pair of very fine forceps, I set about cleaning the skin and abrasions and picking out the larger foreign bodies.

I was somewhere through this tedious process when the attending breezed into the room and said, "What happened here?"

The patient was rather embarrassed and didn't really want to go into an extended version of her history, and so she simply said, "I was running from a 'wolf.'"

The attending physician said, "Where did this occur?"

The patient's reply was "Up the canyon near the restaurant."

The attending physician, deep in thought and without hesitation, said, "There are no wolves in the canyon. Are you sure it wasn't a coyote?"

I felt the patient's embarrassment, and we didn't smile or laugh at the attending physician's ineptitude. I just looked at the patient, shrugged my shoulders, and continued with my work. After removing all the embedded bristles from the patient's skin, I cleaned and dressed the abrasions and set her on her way with aftercare instructions. I realized that that attending physician probably was never going to be very good at bedside manner.

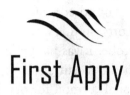

First Appy

When first starting out in practice, the new clinician is making the transition from a teaching center, where older and more experienced physicians have served as mentor, to the real world, where you now make your own decisions, including the decisions about when to consult with others or when to rely upon your own information. Although you have been increasingly accepting responsibility for patients, you are accustomed to the benefit of being able to look to others for the final answer or the *right* way to do things and for the keys to efficiency and successfully practicing medicine. One of the more difficult situations for a physician is when the clinical evidence changes or no longer supports the direction you have been going with a patient's care. That is, you may have made a miscalculation or a mistake, of sorts. Now hopefully, any mistake made is of a minor nature and does not place the patient at significant risk. One experience, gained just after beginning practice, related to these two circumstances.

I was asked, as the newest member of the medical staff, to assist another, more seasoned physician, in fact, the oldest member of the medical staff, on an appendectomy (appy). I followed along for the pre-op visit, where the procedure was explained to the patient, including the operative risks, and the reason for the procedure. I examined the patient's abdomen and found that it was firm, tender, quiet, and showing significant pain localizing to the area of the appendix. The patient's blood count was elevated, and there was no other evidence of an alternate cause for the pain. I agreed that the patient's appendix needed to be removed.

The procedure was begun and proceeded uneventfully to the removal of the appendix. The appendix appeared, however, to be normal. Adjacent to the appendix are some lymph nodes, part of the body's infection fighting system, which were inflamed, enlarged, and likely the source of the patient's symptoms and lab findings. These events occurred prior to the age of widespread imaging of appendices preoperatively to confirm the presence of an enlarged and inflamed appendix. The history, laboratory findings, and clinical exam were used to make the decision. This led to a level of about 10–12 percent false positives. That is, the appendix would turn out to be normal in about 10–12 percent of the cases, even though the patient presented with all the signs and symptoms of an inflamed appendix.

The rationale was that, it was better to be a little bit aggressive and risked taking out a normal appendix than to allow the appendix to quietly fester and rupture, which greatly increases the complication rate of the otherwise simple surgery. Mesenteric adenitis, as this condition is called, was commonly mistaken for a "hot" appendix and was the cause of many of the false positive exams in the past.

So here was the newly trained physician, about to see how an experienced practitioner dealt with the situation of having to tell the family members that the appendix he had removed was, in fact, normal. The surgeon went directly to the family's room, pulled down his mask, and began.

"Everything went smoothly, and he is doing well in the recovery room."

The family asked, "How bad was it? Had it ruptured?"

"No, it hadn't ruptured…but it was completely covered with serosa, and it had a lumen all the way through the middle of it."

Serosa is the name of the thin layer of tissue that makes up the normal lining of intestine, including the appendix, and *lumen* is the term for the hollow center of the tubelike bowel and appendix. So he said essentially, "The appendix was normal," but the family stood in awe of a great practitioner who had rescued their patient from the grips of the serosa and lumen that were afflicting their family member's appendix. And I stood in awe of perhaps the greatest public relations practitioner I had ever seen.

"You're Gonna Love This One"

Taking night call is the bane of the primary care physician. I mean, I know that illness occurs twenty-four hours a day, around the clock, and patients can't always schedule their illness during your office hours. I have seen many illnesses that have progressed along a dangerous path that would have benefited from earlier intervention. That said, there are some cases that could wait until the following day when the office is open. The problem is in telling which is which.

One night, about two in the morning, the phone rang at the head of the bed. I'd learned early on in my career that late-night phone calls were generally for me, so the phone was on my side of the bed. Also, I'm a sound sleeper, so the ring volume was generally up high, to make certain that I heard it. A late-night phone call could be anything: illness, trauma, accidents, anything. Someone would have a question that would, in their mind, be serious enough to look into immediately, and would lead them to call the on-call office number. This would put them in contact with the operator, who would call the on-call doctor. Most often, the operator would ask the nature of the problem, more to make certain that it wasn't just a prank or a common-sense question. So they usually knew what the call was about when they put it through.

This night, when my phone rang, and I put my brain into business mode, the operator simply said, "Dr. Davis, you're gonna just love this one," and clicked to transfer the call to me.

The voice on the other end of the line was a young-sounding mother. I could hardly make out her voice because of the background noise of a vigorously crying infant near the telephone handset. Probably, the child was in the mother's arms as she called me.

I said, wide-awake by now, "This is Dr. Davis. How can I help you?"

She said, "My baby has wet diapers and won't sleep."

I thought, *Wet diapers? Surely, this mother didn't call at two a.m. over a wet diaper. There's got to be more…*

I said, "Is your baby sick?"

She said—baby still crying loudly in the background—"My baby has had a flu bug. He saw the doctor today, who told us to give the baby extra fluids, so he wouldn't dehydrate. I did that. He has wet diapers. He never has wet diapers at night. He has wet diapers and won't sleep."

I said, "Has he got a fever?"

She answered, "No." (baby crying near the phone in the background)

I said, "Any vomiting?"

She answered, "No." (baby crying in the background)

I said, "Has your baby been eating?"

She said, rather frustrated, with the baby still crying in her arms, "I'm sorry, I can't hear you. My baby's crying. I'm going to put him down." At which point, the crying became more distant as she had apparently put the phone down while she walked away with the baby.

Silence on the line.

Suddenly, the phone was picked up, and a gruff male voice said, "Who is this?"

I said, "This is Dr. Davis. Your wife called me about a sick baby."

The voice said, "Our baby's not sick. He just won't sleep…now leave us alone!" and bam! He slammed the phone down.

In the dark, I looked at the phone in my hand, hearing the return of the dial tone to the line.

My wife sleepily said, "Anything serious?" thinking that I may need to get up to go see someone who was ill in the night.

I said, "Um, some people probably shouldn't have kids…"

Patient Honesty

As it turns out in medicine, patients are not always honest with you. Most often, it is purposeful, with the patient having in mind some gain that they believe can only be achieved through dishonesty. A prime example is the drug-seeking patient. In my emergency medicine experience, I've certainly come across my share of those. I learned a very valuable lesson early on in my first few weeks of practice. I was on call in my new community, where call was taken by telephone, from home or wherever, so long as a phone was nearby, and you could respond to the hospital within fifteen minutes.

It was Sunday morning, and my pager beeped, signaling me to call the hospital operator, who served in the capacity of answering service for all the doctors in the community. The operator would either take a message, giving me a number to call back, or if the caller chose, stay on the line, and I would be connected directly with the caller. I called the hospital, and the call was promptly picked up by the hospital operator, who had a caller waiting. The caller gave me his name and told me that he was not a resident of my community but was traveling on the nearby interstate highway. During the car ride, the caller had developed back pain, and over the interval of the drive, the pain had intensified. He felt that he needed some pain medication. He indicated that he was undergoing treatment for cancer and was suffering from pain in a chronic pattern, for which he had been prescribed pain medications. He had forgotten to bring along his medication bottle and needed some medication to control his pain for the duration of the trip. The story sounded reasonable, but it actually wasn't. As we talked, his request grew from just getting enough medication to see him through his trip to providing a month's supply since "he was going to the pharmacy, anyway, and it would save him money in the long run." Also, my concerns were further heightened when he asked for a particular pain medication, a potent narcotic, by brand name, suggesting that other medications would not work for his pain symptoms. I was new to private practice, but I not born last evening. Not only was I concerned about the drug-seeking potential of this caller, I was certainly not going to provide a supply of narcotic medications to someone who was driving a car on the interstate highway.

I listened carefully, asking questions to make certain that he was not having any more serious problems, then assured him that I would provide him a medication that would control his pain. I telephoned the local pharmacy, requesting that they provide the patient with a supply of nonnarcotic pain medication that would be adequate for a week. I guess that word was out that there was a new doctor in town because I had four additional calls within about three hours that morning, all requesting narcotic pain medications. Later in the week, I discussed the weekend's calls with other providers in the community, and they all laughed, knowing that I'd been tested.

S&H Green Stamps

A male physician practicing obstetrics has to learn to overcome many limitations to examining and providing care for the opposite sex. During medical school, the student, both male and female, is required to attend specifically designated courses that are designed to help them overcome any reservations they may have regarding issues of sexuality, gender, reproduction, sexually transmitted illness, and similar topics that they may find troubling. Over the period of my training, I overcame any previous bashfulness or timidity that my conservative rural upbringing may have imprinted into my mind. This, combined with a commitment to listen to my patients as they described their concerns, taught me that the shyness of others may be overcome by a caring manner and gentle humor directed at a patient's own reservations. These principles worked their way into my bedside manner and helped me to develop a large primary care patient population.

One of these patients had come to my office for her annual exam. This type of exam often combined a general health checkup, screening for chronic illness, including cancer, and a consultation about family planning. My usual procedure for one of these exams was to have the patient give samples of blood and urine to the lab on the way in, fill out a health questionnaire to update my records on any problems that may have developed or changed since our last visit. Next, in the exam room, I would review the history and begin the exam, paying careful attention to the head, eyes, ears, nose, throat, lungs, heart, back, spine, and extremities. Then I would give the patient a gown, step out for a few moments, and return with the nurse to examine the breasts, abdomen, pelvic, and reproductive system. This method worked very well for me, giving me a natural break in the middle of these exams, which were of longer duration than my usual office visits. While the patient was changing, I could examine another patient, catch up on phone calls or paperwork or tend to other office duties for a few minutes. Then the nurse and I would reenter the room and complete the exam, with the nurse helping me with the equipment necessary for the exam of the pelvis and collecting the specimen needed for the pap test.

I was at this point in the exam, sitting on a rolling stool at the foot of the exam table, preparing to complete the pelvic exam and pap test when I noticed a small adhesive sticker, the type that children play with, fixed to the inner part of the patient's upper leg. I realized that the patient, sitting in a very vulnerable position, unclothed, recumbent, knees separated, with a member of the opposite sex poised to perform an unpleasant procedure, was not likely aware of the artwork adhering to her inner thigh. Patients in that position generally just stared at the ceiling, and I had a large poster pinned to the ceiling directly over the head of the bed, where their eyes would naturally rest that showed an image of a small kitten hanging from a metal bar by its front paws, with the caption "Hang in there, baby," a reminder of the pop sayings of the early seventies. Occasionally, a patient would prefer to sit in a more upright position, with a pillow under their head such that the examiner could actually make eye contact and carry on a conversation during the exam. But I had long since given up my practice of offering to have the nurse hold a large mirror in a position for the patient to actually watch her own exam, finding that very few patients agreed to participate and some were actually offended at the thought of being able to see the inner parts of their genitalia.

This patient was in the completely supine position, preferring no pillow or upward angle to the head of the table. She couldn't see my gesture then, as I turned to the nurse standing next to me, smiled, and pointed at the sticker. The nurse returned my smile, knowing that I was likely to make light of the situation. I casually reached up, grasped the sticker, and while gently peeling it off her skin, said, "You must have been a very good patient because you got a sticker at the doctor's office."

She leaned up, looking at the sticker stuck to my gloved fingers, and blushed, saying, "Well, if you had any toilet paper in your restroom, I wouldn't have had to use a tissue from my purse. I guess that sticker was stuck to the Kleenex I used."

Chagrinned, I promised that we'd check the paper supplies in the restroom immediately after her exam. We both laughed and continued the exam procedure, the demeanor of the exam room having been lightened extraordinarily and unexpectedly from that point on.

"Hey, Don't Touch My Thingy"

Practicing obstetrics was always one of my favorite parts of practice. I know that it's been occurring regularly for thousands of years before physicians ever ventured onto the scene, but many experiences that I've had in delivering new babies into the world remain some of the highlights of my medical practice. The practice of obstetrics always has the ability to deliver the highest of natural highs and the lowest of lows when things don't go as they should. Sometimes, it is just plain funny. Different women handle labor differently. Some are very stoic, effortlessly managing the contraction pain, pressure, mess, and loss of privacy that may come with the birthing process.

I had one patient in my practice that, for each of her two labors under my care, smiled this beautiful full smile, all the way through her contractions, pushing, the crowning of the baby, and the birth. Others don't handle the discomfort so well. They may even get cross or short with those people who are trying to assist them. One such recollection took place in the labor room. The patient had been admitted in active labor. She was in the part of her labor where the contractions were close together and strong enough to be distractingly uncomfortable. It was not her first baby, so the labor would likely go quickly. She had been placed in a gown, in bed, and an IV line had been placed into her left forearm, near the wrist. This line would serve as a source for the rapid administration of fluids or medications, should the need arise. Otherwise, it just sat there, with the hollow IV catheter inside her vein, and the site protected by tape to hold everything in place. Her husband was sitting, supportively at her left side, holding her hand. I noticed that he was a little nervous, and each time I visited the couple, I tried to reassure them both that things were progressing smoothly, and she should be completely dilated within a short time, and that the baby looked healthy on the monitors. She was monitored with a device that recorded her labor contractions by the tightening of her abdomen registering on a small sensor that was firmly held against her bulging abdomen by an elastic strap. She also had a second sensor against her lower abdomen that recorded the baby's heartbeat. This produced a sound from the monitor that sounded like the rhythmic swooshing of an old-fashioned washing machine. Things looked good. I studied the recording of her monitors and saw a nice, healthy heartbeat and a pattern of steady uterine contractions that registered as a series of "humps" on the monitor paper strip. She had just finished a significant contraction, and I knew that it was time to check the progress of the labor by checking the cervix dilation and confirming the position of the baby's head in the pelvis. That required an internal check. I picked up a single glove from the box and placed it on my hand.

I said rather routinely, "I'm going to check the baby now with an internal check. I don't expect that it will hurt." I placed the gloved hand against her genitalia and started to check for the baby's head position. I was carefully watching what I was doing, checking for any bleeding or the presence of the dark-green stain of meconium, the fluid from the bag of waters that occurs when the baby becomes stressed during labor.

Just then she abruptly and loudly yelled, "Don't touch my thingy!" Startled, I sat back, made eye contact with her, and blushed.

"I have to check on the baby's position," I said, "There really isn't any other way to do it."

Then it was her turn to blush. Her husband, somewhat apprehensive at the whole procedure, had been caressing her arm with his hand. He had chosen that very moment to brush his hand over her IV site and had moved it slightly, causing her some discomfort. She was talking to him, telling him not to touch her IV site and not talking about my exam. That served as a real ice breaker, and things went smoothly from that point on.

Embarrassment Fly Down
Running Injuries

After I had been in practice a while, I had renewed my interest in sports medicine and was serving as the team physician for a local high school. I worked in conjunction with an area orthopedic surgeon (bone specialist) to provide the initial evaluation and referral, as needed, of injured athletes. The orthopedic surgeon was sponsoring an educational meeting for many of the coaches and their staffs, particularly their athletic trainer staffs. The meeting was to be held at a local university lecture room and would be attended by nearly one hundred interested individuals. He asked if I would like to speak at the meeting about a topic, and when I agreed, he assigned me to talk about *running injuries.*

I had given some organized presentations as a medical student and as a resident, but very infrequently, and always as one who was still in training. This time I was to give my talk as a recognized "expert" to a public group and not just to my classmates. I organized a talk of about one hour's length on the topic, prepared my visual aids, handouts, and got a skeleton to demonstrate some anatomic principles to the group. On the day of the talk, I made certain that I had everything ready and then attended all the presentations that were scheduled before mine. I say there was a variety of speaking styles, from droning lectures to exciting demonstrations, including real-patient evaluations right there in the auditorium. Because my presentation included both lecture and demonstrations, I made a mental note to be certain not to be boring and to make liberal use of the demonstrations since they seemed to be more interesting and hold the audience's attention better than simply lecturing. My appointed time was in the slot just after lunch. I finished lunch, stopping by the restroom and then heading to the lecture site.

The room filled rapidly, with people anxious to continue the interesting (so far) conference. I noticed that many of the coaches, particularly the more senior ones, sat in the back rows. To catch a little sleep after lunch, perhaps. That left the front row seats for the younger crowd, the trainers, and newer coaches. A surprising number of them were female, and I made a mental note of that, wondering how the typically shy high-school male athletes that I most often dealt with would do with a female trainer examining them. This was at a time when women's sports were on the increase, following implementation of Title IX, which mandated, among other things, equality in women's athletic programs when compared to men's programs.

I began the talk by reviewing the pertinent anatomy of the foot, ankle, knee, and hip. I was going to concentrate on the foot and ankle since the knee and hip and their related medical problems had their own place on the meeting agenda. I was using photographic slides that I'd made, displayed from a Kodak projector (in the era before power point slide shows, they were known as 2 × 2 slides). I spent part of my time at the dais and part of the time at the skeleton and some other visual aids that I'd brought. The visual aids were located off to the side, so they wouldn't interfere with the audience being able to see the projection of the slides. After a trip or two back and forth, I noticed a group of three young women, trainers, talking among themselves. At first, I thought they were commenting on one of the points of my talk. As time went by, they continued to discuss, whatever it was, much longer than I thought would be necessary in order to gather my ideas. Next, my ego led me to believe that they were, perhaps, talking about me, maybe commenting on my vast knowledge of foot anatomy and the interactions of the bones, tendons, and arches in running. I was just getting to the part about injuries and was certain that they would be very impressed as I outlined all the various problems that could arise with the impact of the heel as it strikes the running surface, the overuse problems associated with workouts, and the various presentations of stress fractures.

It suddenly dawned on me that they were discussing something humorous. Oh, I thought, they'd been enveloped by my charming sense of humor. I stood at the lectern, very impressed with myself, when a horrible thought suddenly entered my mind. What if, no, it's impossible. What if my fly were down? What if I'd returned from the restroom after lunch and started right into my presentation, and all this time my zipper was undone? Well, I was behind the lectern, after all. Certainly I could nonchalantly lower a hand and check, very, very coolly, without drawing any attention. I could do it without anyone even noticing at all. I casually lowered my left hand, as I used my right hand to point at something on the displayed slide. My index finger found the metal teeth of the zipper, and sure enough, the two sides were gaping apart. The fastener was wide open. "Ensign Hanes reporting a hull breech on the lower deck, sir."..."Our next guest is someone who needs no introduction..."

I was horrified. I knew that I must have visibly reddened. I'd bet I was glowing! I finished my point. I knew that I couldn't leave the lectern one more time, now that I knew that it was down. I'd either have to fix it or spend the rest of the talk hiding behind the lectern.

I knew that I had a slide coming up where I'd planned to demonstrate the bony prominences of the foot, showing how the foot was susceptible to injury at the plantar fascia in the arch and that meant leaving the security of my hiding place. *What the heck,* I thought. I just reached down and zipped up, standing as I was in the refuge established behind the wooden lectern. I paused a moment afterward, staring at the young ladies on the front row. They immediately leaned together and began to chat, smiling at one another.

I said, to the group, "You know, I've given this whole lecture to this point, with my fly in the down position. I'm horribly embarrassed, but I have corrected the situation." I continued, "Unfortunately for me, those in the front row noticed it but didn't say anything. I can only assume that it was an error that they preferred go uncorrected." Then "Let's get back to running injuries." I finished up, pretty much uneventfully after that, and received several nice comments about the talk. No comments about the clothing predicament. It's funny, but since that one occurrence, I always check my fly before a presentation. Bad memories really leave a lasting impression.

This wasn't to be my only experience in this regard however. Years later, after I had passed board certification in emergency medicine and was attending a national meeting comprised of practicing emergency physicians and was attending a lecture presented by a world-renowned speaker on the subject of *evaluation of stroke*, the speaker finished talking to the group. He then proceeded to answer questions from the audience and, afterward, walked out of the lecture room with an associate with whom he was having a conversation at the time. The two of them proceeded, apparently to the restroom, without the speaker removing or turning off his still-functioning lapel microphone. This provided much entertainment as the previous speaker's microphone continue to function within the confines of the restroom providing an opportunity for continued amusement of the audience from their conversation. At least my audience was smaller.

C-Section with Bladder in the Way

The practice of medicine is usually a process of repetition, tailored to the specific circumstances of the moment. For example, when performing a physical examination, nearly every person examined has two ears to look into. The anatomy is nearly always the same, and the important aspect of examination is to look for specific things that make that particular ear unique or different. You might see, for instance, scarring or evidence of prior injury to the earlobe. The eardrum maybe scarred or red and bulging in the case of infection. So it is the deviation from the normal that make a physical examination of interest to medicine. It is also the deviation from the norm that can make medicine all too exciting. Most surgical procedures involve tasks that are completed in a particular order, for reasons of patient safety and efficiency. The order for those tasks has long since been established by other surgeons, likely by trial and error, and passed on to new generations of surgeons during training.

I knew that I was not going to be a general surgeon. I came by that knowledge early on in my third year of medical school. However, I still enjoyed surgery and thought that, in order to practice obstetrics in a smaller community, I should have a knowledge of, and skill for, caesarian deliveries. Therefore, during residency, I made a special effort to gain as much experience as I could with caesarians. I would stay late or come in on unscheduled days, just to scrub in on a C-section. During my final year of residency, I made arrangements to be on call at another hospital in town, just hoping to be called to help with case. I received enough experience that I felt comfortable in adding caesarian-section deliveries to my surgical procedure privilege list.

Several months into my practice, I had a patient scheduled for an elective section. That means that she had previously delivered by C-section, and because of the risk of uterine rupture from a subsequent normal labor, she was instead scheduled to deliver by C-section again. The arrangements were all made. Her husband was going to be in the delivery room with her. Because of some bad experiences with her prior deliveries, she was choosing to deliver under general anesthesia rather than stay awake with an epidural or spinal anesthetic. She was going to watch the delivery later by having her husband videotape the surgery. This was not, at the time, an unusual request for a repeat section. The only problem that it presented, really, was the general anesthetic. When moms receive general anesthetic, regardless of the type, they spread it, via their blood stream, across the placenta and into the blood of the baby. Timing is critical because, after a few minutes, the baby becomes sleepy, as well as the mom. What you least want to have, as the product of a delivery, is a sleepy baby. Newborn babies have to cry, to open up their lungs, and to take deep breaths, in order to increase the oxygen content of their blood. It is this increase in oxygen content that causes some of the plumbing connections within the baby's body to switch from fetal circulation to newborn circulation. If this process is delayed or fails, a "blue baby," or a baby with abnormal heart function, can result. The key, then, is to rapidly induce the anesthetic and rapidly deliver the baby, separating the baby from the anesthesia source. I had done this procedure many, many times, both as an assistant and as the primary surgeon.

Everything was ready in the operating room. The staff was present, in their usual places. Soothing music was tuned in on the radio. The baby's bed was ready, with the warmer on to greet the newborn with a nice, soft, warm place to start life. I repeated my usual mantra of the pre-op check list to the scrub nurse.

"Lights, suck, buzz, cut?" which meant, "Are the sterile light handles in place? Is the suction handle and tubing connected and operating? Is the electrocoagulation system on and operating? And is the scalpel ready?"

She nodded. I asked Dad if he was ready, Mom if she was ready, and then I asked if the anesthetist was ready to make the patient sleepy. All systems go. I nodded to the anesthetist, who administered the first of a series of medications aimed at sending the patient into la-la-land. I watched as his thumb pushed the plunger of the syringe all the way down, and he nodded back to me. Lights, camera, action. I made the first incision in the skin, carefully cutting around the prior scar tissue, so that it could be removed, later, in order to make the final tummy scar look better. I entered the subcutaneous tissue with a new, fresh scalpel, deftly slicing down to the layer of muscle beneath it. I carefully opened the muscle by dividing it along the natural lines of separation, making sure to, once again, plan for removal of the scar tissue at the time of closing the incision. I found the peritoneum, the thin lining of the inner compartment of the abdomen, raised it up, making certain that there was no bowel adhering to the under surface from previous surgeries, and up popped the bladder, into my operative field, and blocked my view of the underlying uterus.

"Whoa, what's that bladder doing here?" I asked the scrub nurse. The bladder had popped up into the surgical field, blocking my view of the underlying neck of the uterus. Routinely, the bladder is drained by the pre-operative placement of a Foley catheter, a hollow latex or silicone rubber tube that has a balloon at one end of it. This balloon end is inserted into the urine channel and on into the bladder, where it can serve as a drain for all the urine from the bladder. The balloon is inflated in order to hold the Foley in place, within the bladder. It is part of the routine pre-operative care given to patients who are undergoing abdominal or pelvic surgery. The placement of a Foley catheter was part of my standard pre-op orders.

"The Foley is kinked and isn't draining. Can you unkink it?" I said to the circulating nurse in the room.

Moments were ticking by. The anesthetic medicine was coursing through the veins of the mother-to-be and would shortly be entering the baby's circulation. I got nothing but a blank look from the circulating nurse and scrub nurse.

I repeated my request, "Can you please unkink the Foley catheter?"

The two nurses looked at each other. Then the scrub nurse turned to me with one of those deer-in-the-headlights looks and said, "Foley catheter?"

Oh no, I thought, *no Foley catheter?*

Moments were ticking by. The medications were on their way. The videotape was running. I couldn't proceed because the bladder was blocking my path. This could be disastrous. At first, I thought that placing a Foley now would be an option. However, the patient was on the surgical bed, with equipment trays all around and safely nestled under heavy surgical sterile drapes. Someone, probably the circulating nurse, since she was the only one available, would have to crawl up beneath the poor patient's knees, with a flashlight since it would be pitch-dark under the drapes, and find the urethral opening and insert the catheter. There was no time for that. My mind raced. I quickly asked for a large diameter epidural needle, one usually used for placing an anesthetic deep in the tissues around the spinal cord for aesthesia. I got the needle, attached it to the suction tubing, and carefully pierced the bladder wall. With a relieving sucking sound, the bladder quickly emptied and returned to its position beneath the lower edge of the incision. I was able to insert the retractor to hold it out of the way and proceed with dividing the peritoneum, exposing the neck of the uterus beneath it. The surgical procedure returned to routine once again, but I was still concerned about the baby. Had it gotten enough anesthetic to be born sleepy? Would it need reviving in order to take its first breaths? I spoke to the physician awaiting the newborn, casually mentioning that he would possibly need to be ready for a sleepy baby.

The baby was oriented head down in the uterus. I carefully entered the uterine wall, making sure to protect the baby's head from the advancing scalpel. The bag of waters bulged out at me through the uterine incision. It looked just like the bladder had looked, just a few moments ago. I didn't want to remember that particular image. I stuck it with the scalpel blade, holding the baby's head out of the way. Out came a gush of amniotic fluid, signaling that I was in the uterine cavity. The baby's head had dark hair and was covered with the greasy white material that helps babies stay water-proofed before birth. This made the baby's head slippery and hard to grasp. My heart was pounding, and I was sweating. Moments were ticking by. I lifted the baby's head and face upward and suctioned its nose. It gave a little grimace when I placed the bulb syringe into its nasal passages to clear them of liquid.

That's a good sign, I thought to myself. *Not too sleepy, maybe.*

I delivered the head, then the shoulders, and then the chest, abdomen, hips, and the feet slid out, expelled under the pressure of the reflexive squeezing of the uterus. I clipped the umbilical cord with a plastic clip and clamped a surgical clamp next to it, to allow the cord to be cut without a lot of blood loss. Moments were ticking by. Typically, I'd invite the Dad to cut the cord, but Dad was busy videotaping the delivery, and I wanted this baby to be handed off to the waiting baby doctor as quickly as possible. I grasped the surgical scissors, handed by the scrub nurse, and divided the cord.

"There you go, little one, now breathe," I said aloud, as I handed the baby off to be warmed and to receive some oxygen.

The one-minute Apgar score looked good—a 5 or 6. I thought, *Not bad.* I turned my attention back to the surgical field, where the placenta was making its appearance. I placed clamps at the edges of the uterine incision, to control the bleeding, and delivered the placenta. From the corner of the room, I heard the glorious sound of a small pair of lungs taking their first breaths and bellowing forth with a magnificent and lusty cry. I also heard great sighs of relief from each of the operative team.

The baby doctor turned and said, "Color is good. Lungs sound good, and muscle tone is normal."

All this meant that the baby had been delivered before receiving enough anesthetic to become sleepy. Relieved, I turned to the circulating nurse and said, "Grab a Foley and a flashlight…I've got a chore for you to do." I turned back to the operating table, to the exposed uterus, and began the repair of the uterus. *Just another day at the office,* I thought to myself.

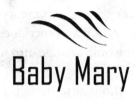

Baby Mary

One of the best stories that I like to tell started out as an uneventful trip to the delivery room for routine OB patient. As I recall it, there was nothing remarkable about the delivery or the aftercare. As I finished writing the delivery note, making sure the mother was properly cared for with orders for meals and medications, I was at the nurses' station making some idle chitchat with the nursing staff when one of the other nurses came out to the desk and said, "Dr. Davis, would you see one more patient for me?" She said, "I know you're not on call, but this lady is from out of town, sees a doctor for her pregnancy that is in OB in the neighboring community, and wants to know if she is in active labor before driving the twenty-five-mile trip to the neighboring hospital."

If I chose not to see the patient, this responsibility would fall to my partner, who was probably home, tucked warmly in his bed or enjoying an evening with his family, which he would have to interrupt to make a special trip to the hospital. As I was already at the hospital, she wondered if would I mind seeing her on his behalf and doing the labor check? I readily agreed to see this patient because we covered for each other in this manner all the time being the small-town medical practice that it was.

Upon entering the room, I noticed two young parents, husband and wife, and noticed that the mother's tummy didn't look very big. I introduced myself and reviewed the history with her quickly and determined that she was nowhere near her due date. I pulled out my OB calendar, which consisted of a circular calendar, divided into forty weeks and printed with month names around the outer ring edge, saw that she was only about eighteen weeks gestation, which seem to fit with her apparent tummy size. I asked her how many children she had; to which, she responded two, then asked her how many pregnancies she had had; to which, she gave the surprising answer of many. As I clarified this history with her, I found that she had delivered two healthy children several years earlier, followed by several miscarriages and at least one stillbirth. She was very concerned about this pregnancy and, as a result, had called her obstetrician when she started to feel cramping in her stomach because she was worried about the possibility of another miscarriage. A brief sterile exam revealed that she was indeed in active labor and already had a fully dilated cervix with active contractions. I immediately placed a telephone call to the closest newborn intensive care, located at my training hospital, and spoke with the neonatologist. Upon learning of her dates and history of complications, the attending gave me the very discouraging news that this was not a viable pregnancy at this time, that the patient would likely proceed with delivery of a nonviable fetus and would suffer the loss of an additional newborn. I asked the second time if there was anything else to be done, such as medication to stop the labor, and he reassured me that it would be ineffective at this point.

Armed with this disappointingly sad news, I returned to the mother's room to present the possible options to the couple. She was already well advanced in labor with a completely dilated cervix, and no way to stop the inevitable delivery. From her reaction, I could tell that she had feared this possibility, and both she and her husband looked at each other hopelessly as I gave in this dismal news.

We prepared the room and staff for the immediate delivery of this premature infant. Within a very few minutes and following a few brief contractions, she expelled the normal-appearing premature male infant, appearing to be about seventeen or eighteen weeks gestation based on the recognizable developmental landmarks, such as palm creases, increases in wrinkling of the skin, and other recognizable indicators. I carefully wrapped the baby in a warm blanket and waited the delivery of the placenta. I administer some medication to further control bleeding and watched as the nurse gently handed the very tiny infant to the mother.

I witnessed the emotional surge that occurred at that time between each young parents. At no time in my practice up to that point had I felt so helpless and disappointed in my medical training. There simply was nothing to be done within the confines of the current level of the advancement within the field of obstetrics to prevent the inevitable loss of that baby's life. Today, as technology allows us to extend the treatments available within the newborn intensive care to an ever earlier age at birth and advancements in the care of high-risk deliveries, there may come a time in the near future where this will no longer be necessary. At this point, however, I was forced to stand by, watching this young premature infant struggled with a few futile gasps, wiggled slightly in his mother's arms, and stopped breathing. I reverently stood by while the mother spent time with her husband and her newborn. When sufficient time had passed, the parents, although not by any means done with their grief, turned to me with questioning eyes.

I briefly counseled the mother that, based on my training, there were likely identifiable causes for her repeated fetal loss and that she should seek further guidance from her obstetrician to work through this problem if she desired further expansion of her family.

From my study and understanding of the physiology of the human female reproductive cycle, I knew that the women's cycle consists of several parts. The first part occurring immediately after menses consisted of a proliferative phase, which was represented by increasing amounts of estrogen within the woman's body. Under the influence of this estrogen, an egg started to develop in the ovary, and this egg was essentially floating within a microscopic pond of estrogen. Under the influence of this estrogen, the thick lining of the uterus entered the proliferative phase and began to thicken and ripen. As the liquid estrogen causes the egg to mature and eventually burst during midcycle, other changes sequentially occurred. At the midcycle, the bursting of the growing egg released a spike of estrogen that signaled ovulation and also led to changes in the remaining cells, or eggshell. These cells remaining behind after the release of the egg are known as the corpus luteum. These cells of the corpus luteum want to produce the hormone progesterone, which accomplishes a couple of things. First, it's associated with the temperature spike, which the woman can use as a sign of ovulation if they are monitoring fertility, and additionally, the progesterone supports the egg during the very early stages of development should fertilization occur. Furthermore, the progesterone causes the tissue of the lining of the uterus to begin to secrete mucus, which will serve as a food supply for the egg and associated structures until a placenta starts to develop. This is called the corpus luteal (white body) or just luteal phase of the menstrual cycle. During this time, the egg travels down the fallopian tube and into the uterus. Under normal circumstances and if sperm is present anywhere in the immediate environment, fertilization can occur, and the resulting fertilized egg uses enzymes to burrow its way into the wall of the uterus, establishing blood supply and the potential for future life. If conception does not occur, the corpus luteum involutes over the next several days, and the thickened uterine lining dies and sloughs off, resulting in the menstrual blood flow. I postulated that it was a problem with this transition from corpus luteum to placenta that caused this patient's problem. She did not have enough progesterone being produced by the corpus luteum to support the development of the pregnancy through the early stages of the placental development resulting in the loss of the products of conception. The fix for this problem would be then to support this stage of the developing pregnancy with additional externally provided progesterone.

I learned that this couple was from a nearby community where he worked as a fireman for ATK, a local concern that built space shuttle booster motors. They were both in good health, and I assured them that they had not done anything improper during the pregnancy to cause this premature birth and that I could see no reason why they could not expect a different outcome with future pregnancies. The premature infant himself appeared to be fully formed with no visible defects. I urged her to return to her obstetrician. In discussing the situation with she and her husband, I mentioned that in some of my previous experience I had had occasion to manage patients with some similar excessive fetal loss. For this reason, I urged her to follow up with her primary obstetrician as soon as possible.

Her laboratory work showed her blood to be stable without excessive loss, and she was discharged that night to return to her home.

I was surprised a few days later to hear from this same young mother, who had some additional questions about the potential medical treatments I had discussed with her for excessive fetal loss. In my subsequent conversations with her, I learned that she had discussed this with her primary care physician, but that he had declined to offer her the suggested medication due to some recent experiences he had had with patients to whom he administered that medication that had resulted in births of children with physical defects. I was aware that this complication could occur with older forms of progesterone supplementation to pregnant women but not with the newer available human form of progesterone that I had been taught to administer during my residency training. For the next day or two, we exchanged phone calls during which I learned that her current obstetrician remained unwilling to take the risks with her receiving this medication because of the concerns regarding the known risks of the older medications. She asked me what I thought her options were, and I could tell that she was a sincere, young woman who felt passionately about her desire to have one more child.

I told her that as long as she was fully informed of the potential risks and benefits and that I would be willing to administer the medication to her because of the proven safety and effectiveness of the newer form of the medication and my experience, although brief as it was, showed successful use in a small handful of patients with similar problems. She agreed to come to my office to discuss this, and I met with her and her husband later that week.

Several weeks later, I saw the patient and her husband in the office for the obtaining of a pregnancy test, which was positive. Because she didn't have any problems with the first several weeks of her pregnancy, we established a care schedule and a treatment program, including progesterone injections to be given regularly starting first at the office and then to be administered by her husband and EMT/fireman. I talked to them specifically about the risks, including prematurity, the potential for birth defects, blood clots, and other complications outlined by the medication package insert. Although

I found her able to fully answer questions about my concerns, I also found that she was very dedicated to having one more child and very tearfully admitted that she was willing to take the risks in order to achieve even the possibility of that benefit. This was a mother who had suffered through multiple fetal loss, pain, and discomfort, and was really dedicated to having one more child. I could tell that no amount of discussion of the potential risks was going to dissuade her from this.

Pregnancy progressed with stability, accompanied by no spotting until around the twenty-second week when she had some signs of early labor. I referred her immediately to her previous OB in the neighboring city, recommending that she have a cerclage, which is a surgical procedure that essentially sutures the cervix with a drawstring in a closed position to serve as a deterrent to premature labor. This obviously prevents a normal delivery because of the presence of suture, and so I knew that we would have to remove the suture prior to delivery. The remainder of her pregnancy was fairly uneventful until thirty-eight weeks gestation. At that time, her mother was visiting from California for the pending birth, and we decided to pick a delivery date, snip the drawstring stitch, and proceed with the delivery.

I saw her in the office that afternoon, checked on the size of the baby in order to assess the potential maturity, and proceeded to remove the cervical suture. She was admitted to the hospital where active labor soon became evident. As she neared completion, we made arrangements for the presence of her husband, as well as her mother in the delivery room. This was one of the most memorable deliveries I had attended. In the room with myself and the delivery room nurse were the father, the mother, and the grandmother. Several close friends and the grandfather were standing by in the waiting room. This delivery was such a happy occasion for all with tears flowing from the mother, father, grandmother, and even the doctor.

One of the advantages of working in a small town was that I truly got to know this couple as well as her parents, their other children, and many of their friends and family. I attended the religious ceremony where baby Mary received her name (named for her maternal grandmother) as well as her baptism, graduation, and wedding. Although I closed my practice in Tremonton and started practicing emergency medicine, I stayed in touch with baby Mary and her family over the years because she married one of the nurse's sons from my emergency room practice.

I also became better acquainted with his family and, over the years, served as a medical advisor during the adoption of the child that they accepted into their home to fill in the gap caused by all those miscarried babies leading up to Mary. Interestingly enough, they adopted a young man who had lost his foot while at the orphanage in a lawnmower accident but went on to become an elite athlete in the National Paralympic program, winning gold medals as a disabled sprinter in several sequential Olympics. Truly extraordinary family.

Aspirated Coin

One case that happened during my years in Tremonton and resulted in learning the lesson that sometimes it's better to be lucky in addition to being good. I was covering the ER one afternoon when a mother brought a small child in, perhaps two years old, with a history of having experienced choking. The story was that the child was in Salt Lake City, was choking in a store, and was taken to a primary children's hospital for evaluation. The mother explained that they had done a chest x-ray as well as blood work and couldn't identify the cause for the child's choking. The mother had been released from the hospital with a copy of the child's x-ray, in case the child experienced any further episodes because of the lack of a firm diagnosis. Apparently, the child had experienced one or two episodes of coughing in the intervening hour that it had taken the parents to drive to Tremonton from Salt Lake City. I saw the child in the emergency department, and he seemed to be in no distress, with clear lung fields. He was generally happy despite the presence of a stranger and was actually a little playful. I pulled the x-ray out of the envelope and popped it into the x-ray view box. Our x-ray view boxes were the type that had a clip at the bottom and a clip at the top, and the x-ray folded into a slight bend when inserting it into the metal edges of the view box. The x-ray view box therefore allowed for the viewing of the x-ray except for the very edges of the film. I was having a hard time finding anything wrong with the child when my evaluation was suddenly interrupted by severe spell of coughing followed by the mother saying, "That's what he sounds like."

It was certainly an impressive cough, and I was immediately reminded of what I hear during the winter months with the development of croup epiglottitis. This finding immediately caused me to focus on potential problems in the child's airway, and I turned to review the film to determine the shape and presence of blockage within the airway. Oftentimes with severe croup, you can see something called steeple sign, which is a narrowing of the child's airway due to swelling from the outside surface of the trachea. There was no steeple sign, and at that point in time, I took the film out of the retaining brackets to look at it more carefully, and I noticed at the very extreme bottom edge of the film a small rounded density, which showed up as a white half circle at the edge of the film. I realized immediately that this was not part of the film itself but rather an aspirated foreign body within the child's trachea. The child continued to cough fairly violently as I reached to my emergency equipment, grabbing a pair of McGill forceps, reached into the trachea of the recumbent infant and carefully removed the nickel.

"That should do it," I said and then ordered a second x-ray, including the whole chest to be certain that there were no additional foreign bodies that had been aspirated. Finding none, I reassured the mother and checked again for any evidence of bleeding or injury within the tracheal area and sent the child out with grateful parents. That day, I learned to carefully read every x-ray all the way to the edge, to always believe the mothers of children when they say they have choked, and that there was still something that could be discovered in a small rural hospital that might have been overlooked by a large urban teaching center. In reality, I truly did count my blessings regarding the fortuitous discovery at the edge of the film and realized that it truly was better to be lucky than good.

Chest Tubes in Chevron Service Bay

One morning while I was on call, I was at the hospital making rounds when the ambulance radio notified me of an incoming call. County dispatch was relaying a message from an ambulance that was located at one of the most distant points in our county and was so far away that it required relaying by the county dispatch base station. The call was for a single vehicle involved in a rollover accident on slippery roads near Christmastime. They gave their location as a point in far western Box Elder County, a little over two hours away from our hospital. I had had very few calls in the past from this area but knew it to be very remote, and I also knew that we were the closest available hospital. The ambulance in this remote part of western Utah was staffed by a nurse who was cross-trained as a first responder/EMT and by a second first responder. Through the dispatch relay, they gave the history of the patient as a young male truck driver for UPS delivery service, who was on his route that morning. I later learned that this individual was well-known to all the residents in that location because he routinely delivered their UPS packages, which was one of the few ways that they could receive goods other than physically traveling the two hours to go to the store. They reported that he was awake, alert, and conscious, but that he had suffered what appeared to be a significant head injury and also had painful ribs and somewhat labored breathing. Neither the basic EMT nor the nurse (who was not currently practicing her nursing) had any advanced airway skills, and so I was immediately concerned about any degradation of breathing ability as well as the potential for complications due to the head injury in the ensuing two-hour trip to the small community hospital that I staffed. I assured them that I would be standing by the radio in order to receive any updates as they progressed on their way to the hospital.

As a little bit more time passed and they were somewhat closer to the hospital using both lights and sirens, they came into radio range by making contact with the repeater station located closer to the hospital. They informed me that the patient's condition had deteriorated somewhat with the onset of delirium, confusion, and a moderate increase in the patient's respiratory rate. I decided to prepare for the possibility of further deterioration of the patient's condition and told the nursing staff to gather some supplies for my jump kit, planning to be ready to respond should the need arise. About ten minutes later, an urgent call came from the ambulance giving the information that the patient was now unable to respond verbally and was experiencing some respiratory distress. I had the charge nurse call the backup on-call doctor and informed her that I would be driving myself out to rendezvous with the ambulance and provide enhanced first response remotely. I relayed this information to the ambulance over the county radio system and ran out to my car with the intention of making the now ninety-minute drive to intercept them as soon as I could. As I walked out to the hospital parking lot, I was happy to see the Utah Highway Patrol officer pulled up behind my parked personal vehicle signal for me to jump in the front seat to accompany him. He told me that he had been monitoring the radio transmissions from both the hospital and the ambulance and would provide red lights and siren for a ride along rendezvous with the ambulance. Prior to leaving the hospital, I also initiated a call to the air ambulance service dispatched out of Salt Lake City and directed them to fly directly to the hospital while I went out with the patrolman to see if I could retrieve the patient. While en route, the officer and I determined that it would be a shorter time to advance care if the air ambulance diverted to the small community of Snowville located in northern Utah along the route planned by the ambulance returning from the scene. As we sped along, the roads were fairly clear in town, but because it was lightly snowing, there was some buildup on the rural highways. It became evident that our three pathways would intersect at the Snowville turnoff and seemed the likely place for the rendezvous between the helicopter, ground ambulance, and highway patrol vehicle. We continued to receive updated reports on the patient as the ground ambulance made its way toward Snowville. When we reached the outskirts of Snowville, the ground ambulance was about ten minutes out, and the air ambulance was about fifteen minutes out. I wondered about where we should transfer the patient, and as we came over a small rise at the outskirts of Snowville, I saw our eventual destination to be the Chevron station at the edge of Snowville. The service station had a parking lot that would be large enough to land the air ambulance and achieve the transfer. As we pulled into the intended destination site, it was lightly snowing, but the air ambulance was continuing on its progress despite the lower visibility and weather. As we pulled up with the highway patrol vehicle, red lights flashing, the service station attendant came out, learned of our situation, and offered the warm service bays of his station as a way to accomplish the transfer without subjecting the patient to cold weather. A few minutes later, the ambulance backed up to the service station bay. The door was rolled up, and the ambulance gurney was lifted out of the ambulance. A quick assessment showed that the patient was no longer conscious, was receiving bag ventilation, had obvious chest trauma, obvious head trauma, and several other visible contusions and injuries. The patient had decreased breath sounds on both sides with a somewhat increase force required to provide ventilation. As the helicopter circled overhead, I made the diagnosis of bilateral chest injuries with pneumothorax based on the mechanism of injury and the decrease in breath sounds on both sides. I quickly placed chest tubes bilaterally, intubated the patient, hyperventilated the patient to reduce the carbon dioxide building up in his body, hoping that this would provide some relief from the increased intracranial pressure of the accompanying head injury. The helicopter touched down, and the flight crew left the rotors running while they quickly entered the service bay to assess the patient. They agreed with the assessment so far, transferred the patient to their own equipment, including oxygen monitor and bag ventilation. They took off toward the trauma center in Salt Lake City with a patient who was still moderately unstable but had been given the best available chance for survival by the combined efforts of the first responders, air ambulance, highway patrol, and rural physician.

Huffing Patient

One patient I vividly recall because of the many lessons I learned from the case was that of a teenage boy brought to the office by his mother because she had discovered him in the garage with a plastic bag containing gasoline vapors from which he was repeatedly breathing in through a process called huffing. This was a popular event in the mid-seventies and was a way for teenagers to experience an artificial high. The practice was somewhat dangerous not only because of the concentrated gasoline vapor that was explosive but also the threat to losing consciousness or ingestion injury from the vaporized petroleum products.

The mother was both concerned for the health effects on her son as well as any of the long-term dangers that might be present from the procedure. I was familiar with the inhalation of petroleum vapors both as a dangerous procedure as well as a way of getting high, and so I proceeded to visit with the teenager about his experience, including the frequency and side effects that he had noted. During the office visit, I had my first experience with perhaps overeducating the patient. I was asking the patient about frequency of his activity as well as the breadth of his experience when I asked him, "Have you huffed anything besides gasoline?"

He replied, "Like what?" and then I made the big mistake.

I said, "Well, such as liquid white out."

The patient looked me wryly and said, "Oh, I didn't know that you could."

I turned red from embarrassment, quickly realized my mistake, turned to the mother, and said, "Forget that I said that," and proceeded on with the rest of the visit, issuing warnings and hoping to suppress any further desire to experiment. I really didn't mean to give the patient any ideas, but sniffing white out was a well-known mech-anism for producing a feeling of elation and disconnection.

I was very careful from that point on to try my best not to give the patient too much information nor to disclose alternate methods by which they might accomplish some damage to themselves.

Trauma Team Setup

Several months after setting up my practice in Tremonton, I became more familiar with the medical community, its strengths, weaknesses, and saw some room for needed changes. This came about because of an event that occurred one day when I was not on call. There was a road accident with fairly significant injuries to the driver that resulted in an ambulance call and the patient being brought to the hospital. One of the older physicians who was covering call that day evaluated the patient very briefly, in the back of the ambulance, ordered the patient to receive some pain medication, and be transferred immediately, still in the ambulance, to a secondary hospital approximately forty miles distant, in Ogden. Now this patient had significant injuries to the pelvis resulting from the accident and was in a lot of pain but would have benefited from further evaluation beyond a cursory look and ordering pain medications. The doctor on call had many years of practice experience but did not have any formal training in modern trauma care and therefore sought just to keep the patient comfortable during the transport process and referred to a higher level of care.

This created several problems for the patient because the injectable pain medication carries with it the potential for dangerously lowering blood pressure, adding to the already existing shock of the accident and its accompanying reduced blood circulation. Moreover, pelvic injuries are notoriously associated with large amounts of blood loss, which further increases the risk of hemorrhagic shock. The modern method of treating this patient would involve stabilizing the patient with large-bore IV access, replacement fluid administration, stabilization of the pelvic bones, and then followed by rapid transport to a larger center. Apparently, the ambulance stopped at the next hospital en route to Ogden and requested that they start an IV line to give the patient some fluids and then completed the transport to the larger center. Unaware of these circumstances, I received a telephone call later that morning in my office that began with the statement, "Jim Davis, what the heck are you doing up there?" This was the receiving surgeon from the larger hospital, actually my training facility, stating that he just received the patient with a pelvic fracture who was unstable at transfer and needed fluid resuscitation prior to being taken to the operating room. He said that he had hoped he had trained me better than that and that I should be held to a higher standard than he was seeing when it came to patient care. I told him I didn't know the facts regarding the case, but that I would do some immediate investigation and get back with him.

Due to some experiences of a physician in the Midwest, involving an orthopedic surgeon and his family who were traveling when they experienced a motor vehicle accident with severe injuries, this surgeon experienced firsthand the difficulties and variances currently existing in the trauma care system that prompted him to do research on possible methods of improving care and outcomes. A newly developed program in advanced trauma life support had sprung to life and had begun being taught to orthopedic surgeons, general surgeons, and other interested physicians. This course, known as ATLS, was the equivalent to the American Heart Association's ACLS classes and were meant to prepare physicians, especially rural physicians, for advanced care of trauma patients. Now, as part of my training, I had gone through this course and knew that our local hospital could provide better trauma care than had been experienced by this patient with a hip fracture.

At our next staff meeting, I came prepared with a synopsis of the trauma course and had devised a plan for implementation of a trauma team for our local medical staff. My proposal included a team approach to the evaluation and management procedures as well as a policy for when the trauma team would be called into action and the parameters for selection of patients who would be trauma team candidates. We decided on several triggering events, any one of which could be individually responsible for summoning the trauma team. They included the patient with ongoing loss of consciousness, a patient with multiple significant injuries, multiple patients arriving at the same time, as well as accidents involving significant blood loss in the opinion of the receiving physician. The trauma team would consist of automatically paging at least two physicians, one for supervising the care of the victim and another for actually providing the care or any needed procedures involved in the resuscitation. Additional staff would include the hospital nurse anesthetist, the operating room scrub nurse, laboratory, and radiology who would be automatically called in every situation of a trauma team activation. It was hoped that this would result in sufficient staffing to provide adequate sets of hands for all necessary procedures as well as automatic consultation between multiple care providers for an immediate second opinion in such situations. At our small hospital, it was not our intention to provide the services of trauma surgeons but rather placement of central lines, stat blood draws, and other immediate first-aid stabilization.

At that initial staff meeting, there was actually some dissension expressed from a couple of the older physicians in the community. One of them said, "Well, there's nothing we really can do for these people, and they're leaving town anyway, so why should we try?" Another expressed an unwillingness to be on call anymore often than he was already required to be on call for our emergency room services. The remaining physicians agreed that we would implement the planned trauma team and provide the necessary services with those of us on the staff who were willing to voluntarily provide such services. I reported the results of the staff meeting back to my training surgeon, and he readily commended our efforts in improving the perspective trauma care for patients who came through our emergency room.

We had set up our hospital pagers with a special code that could be used to summon the trauma team when needed. This audible tone was different from a regular pager tone, and we had all agreed to immediately respond to the hospital upon hearing that coded tone. We agreed to respond even if there might be some doubt as to the necessity of the whole team responding with the idea that anyone who is not needed or considered "extra" could return home. Over the time that I remained in that community, prior to taking my board certification in emergency medicine and changing my practice site to Logan Regional Hospital, I saw many instances of successful implementation of the trauma team. The addition of this team approach to stabilization and critical care of our northern Utah patients resulted in lives saved, pain and suffering reduced, and better patient outcomes across the board.

One of the first such activations of the trauma team involved an early morning trauma team call due to a commercial bus rollover on a slick, rain-coated highway north of our community at a place called Rattlesnake Pass on the interstate highway near the Idaho border. This bus was carrying a church group of young teenage boys and girls on their way to a several-day youth conference. When the hospital received the call, they activated the trauma team because there were sixty-three inbound patients, mostly minor injuries, but the trauma team was called because of the overwhelming nature of the patient load. As I recall, there were multiple bumps, bruises, cuts, and scrapes that our medical staff, doctors, and nurses all screened, treated, reassured, and discharged. While this took our medical staff the whole morning to work through, it was not required that we transfer any of the patients outside of our facility for care. We did contact adjacent hospitals to advise them of the situation just in case, but transfer was not required.

Stinky Springs Rollover

Another trauma team call one Saturday night involved some local teenagers who were headed out to a regional hot springs known as Stinky Springs, which was located west of town in a pond of warm water resulting from an active geological site related to the nearby presence of Yellowstone Park. This occurred in the cold dead of winter, and apparently, the teens were planning to skinny dip and were in the process of changing into their swimsuits inside the car when the driver lost control of the vehicle, rolling into the ditch, and injuring some of the passengers. The trauma team response brought enough hands to sort through the mostly-naked victims, including a couple of teenagers, partially dressed in firemen's jackets, who were embarrassed but otherwise not seriously injured.

Another trauma team success story involved a one-car rollover in which the driver was seriously injured by being ejected through the back window of a small compact hatchback vehicle, resulting in a deep, broad laceration to the patient's neck. This, of course, resulted in significant bleeding, shock, and impairment of the airway. I saw my skilled anesthetist insert the endotracheal tube into the patient's airway by following a stream of bubbles emitted by the partially severed trachea. I watched this unfold as I stood beside him at the head of the bed, directing the remainder of the trauma team. This amazing feat combined with the other resuscitation efforts provided by the team certainly resulted in saving that young adult's life. I was truly rewarded, later on, when that young man came to my office to thank me and other members of the trauma team for their efforts.

Most of the times that the trauma team was activated involved major traffic accidents occurring on the adjacent interstate highway in northern Utah. One unusual case of trauma team activation occurred

212

one night when I was on call and had just finished seeing a patient in our local emergency room when a patient entered the emergency room entrance and told the admitting nurse that she was in labor. There was, of course, more to the story. The patient had experienced spontaneous rupture of the bag of waters, followed by the presentation of the umbilical cord, which had prolapsed. This is a very dangerous situation and has resulted in the stillbirth of many, many infants. That night, however, the trauma team was called in response to this prolapsed cord and resulted in the successful delivery of that infant and a healthy, viable start to its life. Because of my training, I knew that the immediate treatment of a prolapsed cord was to place the patient supine, get the head tilted downward in Trendelenburg position, insert a Foley catheter, and inflate the bladder with saline in an attempt to decompress the pinched umbilical cord against the edge of the pelvis. This maneuver resulted in spontaneous return of pulsations to the cord and allowed us several extra minutes with the rapidly assembling trauma team staff to do an emergency C-section, allowing the delivery of a healthy infant. The nurse on duty in the ER that night immediately prepared the operating room, and when the trauma team arrived, it included the operating scrub nurse, a circulating nurse, the anesthetist, as well as laboratory staff and others. Of course, I was already there and performed the C-section, initially under local anesthetic until the anesthetist arrived to adequately sedate and anesthetize the patient. Due to the nature of the small town where we lived and the proximity of the staff and some driving that exceeded the local posted speed limits, I was certain, we were able to deliver that baby within ten minutes of her arrival at the hospital. I was very proud of our staff and team at that result.

Head-On Collision

One other case that I particularly recall had a great unplanned impact on my life and future career. One Thursday evening, my trauma pager went off, and I was informed by the nurse that the team was being summoned to the hospital for a two-car accident with multiple victims, and in addition to a fatality, one of the passengers had suffered a traumatic amputation of the leg. The ambulance radio said that they were en route to the hospital and would be arriving in a few minutes. I lived on the street that was a direct route to the hospital, but to get there, I had to cross the set of railroad tracks that consisted of a slight rise in the street, followed by a return to level, which always created a bit of a bump as I passed that railroad crossing, like a scene from *The Dukes of Hazzard.*

As I arrived at the hospital and ran down the entry hallway, I saw the team members arriving and assembling into their assigned positions. As I was the first to arrive, I took the patient with the reported amputation of the leg. I spoke to the initial first responder who, upon extrication of the victim, had determined that it was not an amputation but rather an open fracture of the lower femur with the leg having been folded down, not initially visible from outside the car, and having the appearance of an amputation. There was, nonetheless, significant blood loss from the open fracture and other injuries. I could tell that this patient was going to need expert orthopedic care in order to salvage the extremity, and so I had the nurse begin the process of arranging for immediate transfer by air ambulance to a larger level 1 trauma center in Salt Lake City. Myself and other team members then proceeded to stabilize this patient by the administration of fluids in large quantities, placement of a hare traction device on the injured leg, and provided primary care for his other injuries. He initially did not have any pulse in that leg, but with the placement of the traction, I was gratified by the return of the pulse. I administered pain medication for his comfort and had the nurse begin to monitor him for stability. I turned my attention to the other victims of this accident to see if I could help with their stabilizing care.

The story, as related by the emergency medical technicians, was that a car containing four high school students from a neighboring school district had come to the local golf course in order to practice their golf game for a tournament that was to occur the following day. They had completed their practice rounds and were in the process of driving down Main Street on their route out of our community when, in the bright setting sun, an eastbound car had struck head-on against a westbound car that had been obscured in the bright glare of the sun.

This was a very challenging accident due to the presence of multiple victims, the seriousness of the mechanism of injury, and the presence of a fatality. The other driver had struck his chest against the steering wheel and had suffered a large bruise across the anterior chest, which had resulted in a contusion of the heart that led to cardiac arrest from *comotio cordis*, which is a rare complication of blunt chest trauma. This patient did not respond to multiple attempts at cardioversion and succumbed to his injuries.

The others injured in the accident, though less severely, remained stable and were treated and released. The air ambulance arrived and received the stabilized patient by way of a "hot load," which is where the arriving air ambulance did not fully shut down its motor but immediately prepared for liftoff for the return flight. I was able to accomplish this by use of a trained and prepared staff who had everything ready at the time of the patient handoff. I realized that local trauma care had been greatly improved in our community by the training and assembling of this remarkable team.

I made daily calls to check on the status of this injured young man. I learned that he was doing well and that his surgeon was able to stabilize the fracture, saving the leg from amputation. As further time passed, I learned more about each of these individuals involved in the accident. I followed the care of the driver, until his release from the hospital, by regular phone calls to the trauma center. It turned out that, in addition to being an avid golfer, he was a varsity basketball player. The following year, when his high school team played our local team, I had the pleasure of meeting him in the visiting team's locker room, where I introduced myself as "the doctor who took care of you during your accident."

I also had the pleasure of meeting his parents after that game, and they thanked me greatly for the stabilizing care provided at our first meeting. It turned out that his mother worked as a nurse and, small world that it is, later became my administrative nurse at the University Health Center, where I completed my career following my experience in primary care and then emergency medicine. One of the great pleasures I have had in my career was getting to know patients, beyond the history and physical and treatment that is brought about by their injury, illness, or other medical need. Some truly lasting relationships had been developed as a result of these diverse experiences.

The Rest of the Story

In a strange twist of fate, I learned an amazing bit of information about my premedical decision while attending that chemistry class at that college in Western Illinois. I was just finishing up seeing a patient and making rounds at the Tremonton Hospital one evening and stopped at the nurses' station to chat for a while with one of the clerks who was getting ready to leave, with her husband, to be a mission president on an LDS mission to Chicago. Because Chicago was my wife's hometown, I wanted a little more information about where they would be and what they would be doing. Her husband, as it turned out, was a high school science teacher, and in a casual way, I asked her who would be teaching his classes for him during his leave of absence.

She replied with the question, "I don't know. Why, do you want to?"

I revealed that I had always had aspirations to teach science, particularly chemistry, at the high school level. She paused and looked at me quizzically saying, "What caused you to give up that aspiration?"

I began my reply with "Well, there was this PhD candidate in *Life* magazine who couldn't find a job."

The nurse standing next to us overheard this conversation and interjected, "Yeh, do you know who that guy was? It was my husband, Mitch."

In a strange twist of fate, I learned that the student that I learned about in chemistry class was, in fact, a graduate student at Utah State University. Moreover, he was actually a patient of mine. After learning of our serendipitous common experience, she brought in a copy of that *Life* magazine to show it to me. As it turned out, I had just seen her husband, the chemist and my patient, with a sprained ankle a week or two previously in my office. What a small world it is!

The world is an amazingly small place indeed. And I can only imagine that somewhere, the Great Creator sees this as something like a scene from *The Wizard of Oz* where the small dog, Toto, pulls the curtain back on the wizard and exposes to the unintended observer what is really going on behind the scenes.

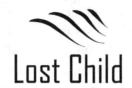

Lost Child

One of the characteristics of a small-town practice is the way in which the physician becomes integrated into the community. This began to manifest itself once I moved from my training center and Ogden, to the site of my first practice in Tremonton. As I settled into the start of my first job, as a practicing physician, my new partner announced his departure on a well-earned vacation about two weeks after my start date. This trial by fire led to my perception of being readily accepted into the community, even being offered a position of honor in the first parade of the summer season, where I served as the driver (probably due to the availability of my convertible sports car for the parade) for a young lady who was part of the homecoming royalty from the local high school.

Over the next several months, I became busier in my practice, and my partner and I reached the point where we were going to build a new building, and I was ready to build a newer, larger home for my wife, who had endured so much during my training years. We got the home built, and I was there, enjoying an evening off with my family, when the doorbell rang. The person at the door informed me that she was a member of a local church group who had received the assignment to distribute flyers to each home in the neighborhood regarding a lost child. I looked at the photo on the flyer and immediately recognized the face of one of my own patients, a five-year-old whose residence was several blocks away from my new home. The story, related by the young woman, was that the child had been abducted from the grade school in our neighborhood. The event had occurred just that evening, and many in the community were involved in the door-to-door canvassing for the lost child. I agreed to help and went over to the school, where the volunteers were assembling, and entered the search. Throughout the evening, we searched the outdoor areas of the school, nearby homes, and any other areas as directed by the local police department and deputies.

Search canines were brought in to aid in the search but didn't seem to pick up much of an identifiable scent. After a few hours spent in this activity, word came to the deputies directing the search that the child had been seen in a community many miles to the north, in the company of an elderly man. Eventually, the little girl was let out of the vehicle and found her way to a rural farmhouse where she had asked the owners of the home to help her. This led to the little girl being taken to the local sheriff's office, who initiated a call to the local peace officers here stating that the girl had been found. Much joy and elation was shared by, of course, the parents, but also the community at large, who had been actively searching throughout the evening.

My own involvement in this case continued, however. As it turned out, I was the primary care physician for this patient, so I knew her parents well and, in fact, had evaluated the child in my office a few weeks previous. In discussion with the sheriff's department, they were making final arrangements for the trip to the distant community to pick up the child. Of course, the concern of the parents and the peace officers was the question of whether or not the child had been assaulted or injured during her abduction. She was reportedly in no distress and had no concerns expressed at the time of her showing up at the farmhouse, but the question remained. As it turned out, the emergency room located nearest to the farmhouse where the child had ended up was one that I had worked in, for many weekend shifts, during my residency, and I still had active privileges at that facility. It was therefore suggested and, I agreed, to travel with the local deputy representative on his trip to retrieve the child and accompany him, along with the child's parents, and to offer the examination of the child within the emergency department located there, should there be any question as to physical injury suffered by the child.

It turned out that the abductor was an elderly man, who put the child in the front seat of his car and drove almost immediately out of town, which was why there were no local signs of the child and no trail to be followed by the search dogs. The other fortunate result of this bizarre event was that there was no evidence of physical injury of the child and no physical evidence to be collected whatsoever, except for some dog hair found on the child's clothing from her contact with the car seat. All this evidence was gathered, given to the police, and the child was joyfully reunited with her parents.

Unfortunately, nationwide, not every child abduction resulted in this type of happy ending. I was grateful for the opportunity to serve the community in this capacity, using my pediatric experience as well as my attachment to the community to be of service to this family in this rather unique way. As I looked back on all the demands placed upon a family physician in a small town, this reminded me of the service element included in nearly every experience I had in that practice setting.

Spence

One unusual case came about one Sunday afternoon when I was on call. I got a call from the hospital operator telling me that one of the local highway patrolman wanted to contact me and the operator was requesting permission to give my home phone number. Now to be honest, my phone number had always been published, but even at that, it shouldn't be too hard for a patrolman to obtain my home number whether for official business or not. This, however, turned out to be "official" business. It seemed the officer was on duty, in a highway patrol vehicle, which required long periods of sitting, and he reportedly had developed perirectal pain from a thrombosed hemorrhoid while on shift that afternoon. He was asking for advice as to whether or not he should come to the ER with that sort of problem or whether I'd be willing to see him in the office instead.

Now here's a little more information about the relationship between law enforcement and emergency department physicians. Our paths certainly crossed at frequent intervals, and we got to know each other pretty well, whether it was providing care for motor vehicle accident victims, patrolman and their families, or just the passing of friendly jokes while waiting for time to pass in the ED. I learned early on in my career, as the reader would recall from the bee incident, that it frequently paid off to know the local law enforcement officers and that included the highway patrol. I'm happy to report that most of my experiences were very positive, and I don't mind at all when I look in my rearview mirror and see that one is following me. I've even been the recipient of some "selective enforcement" due to my relationships that develop in the emergency department.

This day, I agreed to meet the officer in my office to see the nature of the problem. At the appointed time, he walked into my office in full uniform and said, "I think I'll need an exam." We then went to an exam room where I asked him if he needed a gown or not. He reached down to his utility belt, but first, removed his service revolver, placed it on the mayo stand adjacent to my exam table, and said, "Now we're not going to hurt each other, are we?"

I very uneasily replied, "Well, I'm not planning on hurting you...much."

The examination showed that he did indeed have a thrombosed hemorrhoid, which was producing a lot of discomfort as he rode around in his police cruiser. It was a simple procedure to anesthetize the bulging black-and-blue mass, make an incision in the skin down the length of the bulge, and shell out the clotted blood contained in the hemorrhoid. This incision let the edges fall back together and did not require any further closure. There was no active bleeding, and his pain was immediately reduced. Once again smiling, he thanked me profusely and asked about charges. I reassured him that it was professional courtesy from one pain in the butt to another. On other occasions, I used my relationship with this peace officer when I had an emergency that required the timely presence of an out-of-town consultant to help me with an emergency surgery when I had started care on a lacerated foot of a young child and discovered to my dismay that the flexor tendon was involved in the deep reaches of the wound and called on an orthopedic surgeon to assist me with the further repair of that toe. I called the county dispatch, identified the officer who was patrolling the road, and asked that he watch for the passage of the orthopedic surgeon and assist in whatever way he felt necessary. This kind of relationship also led to this officer calling me in the wee hours of the morning one weekend night to assist with the stabilization of a patient involved in a rollover accident down a ravine a few miles out of town. After arriving at the scene, I was asked to make my way down a rope to the location of the search and rescue team at the bottom of the ravine. I assisted in the stabilization of the fractures there in the field, starting an IV for fluid administration, and administering some pain medication from my jump kit carried for just such circumstances. After I completed the round-trip back up the rope and was watching the extrication of the injured driver, this same highway patrol officer asked me with a huge smile on his face, "Did you see any rattlesnakes while you were down there?"

I replied, "No, thankfully."

To which, he began to laugh, stating, "Well, they were all over." It was with this type of professional relationship that I was able to successfully build my practice and survive those early years in the real world.

Baby for Blanket

My practice experience in Tremonton was, for the most part, extremely positive in that I had an enjoyable practice, a good family life, strong friendship bonds, and a continual sense of having a positive impact on the community. The interaction that I had with my patients in that community remained memorable. I always tried to be of benefit and service to my patients, my partners, and the hospital staff. For the duration of my practice, I didn't ever really find myself in a situation where I did not feel justifiably compensated for the work that I was doing. Over the time of my practice, there I performed care consisting of general medical care, surgical procedures, delivery of babies, sports physicals, and other services without counting nickels and dimes. Our office had a low-key approach to collections, which kept us in good standing with the mostly rural and conservative community.

One event that occurred in our community was when a local entrepreneur ran into financial problems, fell behind in his IRS payments, and found that he suddenly needed to change locations to the US Virgin Islands because it was located offshore. Several of his employees were among my patients, including a young mother-to-be who was entering her second trimester of pregnancy when she discovered that she would no longer have coverage by her health insurer due to nonpayment of premium. She came to my office to discuss this, and I assured her that it would be no problem. We would make arrangements to continue her care, uninterrupted, and that I would relieve her from the burden of having to pay for the delivery. I also set up an appointment for her to talk with a financial counselor at the hospital making arrangements for the hospital portion of the care. I didn't think anything more about this until, a few weeks after her delivery of a healthy baby boy. She came to my office and presented me with a beautiful handmade blanket that she had constructed for my benefit. I was amazed at the quality of the handiwork and expressed this to her along with my appreciation for her consideration. My daughter liked the softness and fuzzy feel of that handmade quality item so much that it quickly disappeared into her room, and she has it to this day in her collection of mementos.

Transition from FP to EM

After experiencing the day-to-day medical practice of a small-town environment, I began to look at my practice and what it was becoming with a more critical eye. I was becoming very busy, in part, because my practice was growing, and in part, because I was feeling a growing desire for more opportunities to provide acute care rather than chronic care. Now there were many aspects to my practice that I really enjoyed. Specifically, I loved providing prenatal care, delivering babies, and taking care of children. I wasn't very good at, nor did I enjoy the other end of the age spectrum, such as visiting nursing-home patients. I enjoyed my surgical practice and was very careful to limit to the procedures for which I had received good training and experience. I enjoyed the occasional opportunity to assist visiting surgeons and continued to provide that assistance upon request.

My life was changing, requiring more and more time spent away from home and my children. I remember wondering how I would ever be able to, when the time came, help coach one of their amateur sports teams, attend a dance recital, or spend quality time with my ever-growing family. I began to experience interruptions in my planned vacations and other planned family activities. Additionally, my expanding job activities were mirrored in the lifestyle of my partner, who was experiencing the same complications of his own family life. I was really taken aback when, after about six years of an even busier practice, he announced that he was leaving our practice to go to the island of Guam and continue his practice there. His rationale was that he found his practice to be all-consuming and was interfering with his ability to spend time with his children. Over the next several weeks, I contemplated my future, knowing that I would likely need to make some changes upon his departure.

Our family had already started a new home, and it was at the basement wall stage. We thought briefly about walking away from the construction but decided to continue building while we considered our options. Easy options included contacting some of my previous classmates, who were now in practice in various communities around the state, and see if there were any opportunities available. I even visited a couple of sites distant to my current practice in order to check on possible opportunities. The biggest concern I had was the degree to which my practice had intruded on my personal life and time off. I didn't expect a life of leisure, and I was certainly willing to dedicate a lot of time to the practice of medicine, but many times, this became overwhelming. I would get up each morning and be at the hospital at 6:45 a.m. in order to start rounds or do a scheduled surgery case at seven o'clock. This would be followed by going to the office, from the hospital, and taking whatever lunchtime I could find and working until 5:30 p.m. or 6:00 p.m., by which time, a patient or two had presented to the emergency room at my hospital due to the lateness of the hour and expected closure of the office. My office was located immediately adjacent to the hospital, so while it was only a few steps out the back door between the buildings, it meant that I had a difficult time getting away. I realized that this was a situation of my own creation, but I had recognizable difficulty in extracting myself from commitments either real or perceived to this patient population.

I had several discussions with the hospital administrator regarding some ideas I had to share about how to "turn down" my practice a little and spend more time away and not be on call. The market area for our hospital was about fifteen miles away from a slightly larger hospital, who served as our major competitor. On many, many occasions, I received phone calls in the early evening hours, having just arrived at home, to learn that I had one of my patients in the local emergency room requesting for me to see them. If I replied that I was unavailable, their most likely response was that they would leave my hospital and go to the competing site to be seen. While I enjoyed the attention and notoriety, I continually sought a solution to this problem. I knew it would only get worse with the pending departure of my partner. One event that helped in my decision was that I found myself at the hospital one Wednesday morning and did not see my children awake for the remainder of that week until Sunday night.

A few weeks passed, and I found myself on a Saturday morning needing to consult with a specialist at the regional hospital about a patient with an uncontrolled nosebleed. I called the regional hospital emergency department and asked for the doctor of that specialty who was on call. The nurse answering the phone gave me the doctor's name and then continued, "Jim, have you ever considered doing emergency medicine full-time?" Now recall, I had practiced at this emergency room site during my residency years. A group of doctors at that hospital had recently left their practices in order to practice emergency medicine full-time.

At first, I said, "No, I don't think—" But then stopped and said, "yes, maybe I would consider that." She gave me the phone number for one of the principals in the emergency room group, and I agreed to contact him.

Over the next several days, we met and enjoyed dinner and a description of the practice. I was definitely interested but had some apprehension as to whether or not I could adapt my family-medicine experience to the largely unknown world of emergency medicine. Complicating this decision were the issues surrounding the closure of an active OB practice, reassignment and dispersal of my patient population in a manner that would not leave them feeling abandoned, and embarking on the practice with new partners in emergency medicine. As it turned out, there was a window of time where my boards in family medicine would enable me to also sit for the boards in emergency medicine. This would allow me to become board-certified in both specialties, which I felt very strongly about.

I started picking up emergency department shifts while I simultaneously downsized my practice in preparation for closure. I delivered all my then-scheduled obstetrical patients, hired a new physician to take my place in the community, and began the transition to full-time emergency medicine. As it turned out, there were many similarities between emergency medicine as it was practiced in a smaller urban-hospital setting and its cousin, family medicine. As it turned out, a lot of emergency medicine was simply unscheduled, episodic, primary care. So for this type of practice, I was very well-prepared. Nonetheless, I still found myself very apprehensive during those first few shifts in the emergency department. I found myself faced with new nursing staff, new patient problems for the most part, and a relatively unknown consulting staff. I worked very diligently over the next few months to integrate myself into each of these groups, trying to come to peace with my new home.

From Which Patient Did This Urine Sample Come?

Teasing is one of my strongest characteristics. I believe that it stems back to some early childhood experiences as an apprentice in learning art of teasing from a master teaser. Yes, if he had participated in a medieval teasing guild, he would have easily qualified as a master teaser. It's my burden, and I bear it well.

So it was a typical Saturday morning in the ED, not too busy and cruising right along. Among others in the ED at that time were a couple of young men: one, in his midthirties, who had been out, with a companion, black powder hunting; and the other, a seven-year-old with diarrhea for a week. Black powder hunting is a trip back into history for avid hunters, wherein they hunt game (deer, in this case) with a rifle that functions without manufactured bullets. The rifle is fired by pouring a set quantity of black powder into the barrel, placing a cloth patch in the barrel, and following the patch with lead ball or lead bullet, often handmade. The powder, patch, and shot are then hand-packed into the barrel with a tamping rod, just like in the old days. All this adds to the challenge of hunting big game by giving the hunter only a single shot with older and less-accurate technology. The powder is ignited by a flint/steel spark at the breech of the rifle. The loading process is somewhat time-consuming and does not lend itself to easy unloading of the rifle, if it is not fired. This morning, a pair of black powder hunters had been out in pursuit of their deer. At the first site, they saw no deer and, after a while, decided to move to another site. One of the pairs placed his loaded rifle in the gun rack, above and behind the bench seat of the pickup. Apparently, the flintlock was still in the cocked and ready-to-fire position. His partner got in the passenger side of the pickup and sat back, bumping the rifle with his head. The rifle slid off the gun-rack hooks and discharged, the ball striking the passenger in the neck at close range. The patient arrived in the ED awake, alert, but unable to move his arms or legs, and showing no sensation below his fourth cervical (neck) vertebra level. The nerves from this area go to the upper parts of the chest and back and upper arms. He could still breathe, think, and talk, but couldn't voluntarily move. He was stabilized with an IV, analgesic medications, and a cervical immobilization collar. The x-rays showed that the round shot was not embedded in the soft tissues of the neck, having passed completely through the skin and soft tissues, without stopping or striking any bones. "Just a flesh wound" was the mountain man's response when shown the x-rays. Yet he was still paralyzed from the injury. I suspected that he had suffered *cord shock* from the impact of the bullet. This is a soft-tissue pressure injury that leaves the nerves temporarily nonfunctional, but the prognosis is good that some or all the function will return. I consulted, by telephone, with the regional trauma center and their neurosurgeon, Dr. Church. I knew him from my days of training at the trauma center, and he gave me an optimistic outlook for this patient's course. The patient was stable at that point and awaiting the results of some more of his labs, which included routine things like baseline blood work and a urine test, which would be useful for those taking care of him in the hospital later on. I got him ready for transfer and went on to see other patients while awaiting the ambulance that would transport him to the regional center.

Which brings me to the case of the young man with the diarrhea? He had increasing quantity and frequency of stools over the week but had seen no blood or signs of infection in the stool. He was from a rural area, and his family got their drinking water from a private well, not uncommon in the rural areas of this state. No other members of his family were suffering from similar complaints, which lessened the likelihood of a water-borne or food-borne illness.

One of the problems with diarrhea is that patients lose fluids and become dehydrated, particularly in a desert. An easy way to determine the status of a person's fluid surplus is to look at a urine sample. The kidneys conserve water when the body needs it, by making the urine more concentrated. Likewise, when water is present in abundance in the body, the kidneys will make more diluted water, ridding the system of the excess. Urine concentration is measured by a parameter called specific gravity and can vary in value from 1.000 (very dilute, pure water) to 1.035 (very concentrated.) So I ordered urine test on the child with diarrhea, as part of his workup.

A little later, after the gunshot wound had been transferred, I saw a little plastic cup, with a screw-on plastic lid, on the countertop at the nurses' station—a urine cup, full of urine. It was unlabeled. Now good, careful medicine would indicate that anytime anyone collects a specimen for the lab, they should label it with the patient's identifying information. This prevents lab errors and prevents delays in getting lab results back. Here was an opportunity to do some teaching about good lab procedure and to have a little fun teasing the nurses at the same time. I went to the storage cupboard and retrieved an identical, new, sterile plastic urine cup, and went to the refrigerator in the lounge and got some apple juice. I filled the urine cup about two thirds full of apple juice and took it back to the nurses' station, replacing the unlabeled urine container with the unlabeled apple juice cup. Soon the nurses returned to the nurses' station, and I asked, "Here's an unlabeled urine specimen. Who do you think it belongs to—the gunshot guy or the diarrhea kid?" Neither nurse knew for sure where the sample had come from. I unscrewed the lid and said, "Well, if it's the gunshot-wound guy, I should be able to taste the black powder," and took a big swig. Both nurses gasped. The looks on their faces were priceless. The only bad part was that nurses tend to hold grudges and would go to great lengths to get even.

Doc, I Broke My Dick

One of the things that good practitioners realize at some time during their practices is that there are individualized requirements from each of our patients. Even though the disease is the same, the evaluation and treatment and needs of the patient are different from any other patient seen before. The science may be well established, but the art is different in each case. For a strep throat, the patient could just as easily (and may, indeed, do so in ever-increasing instances) punch a code into an ATM-like machine, and receive the appropriate dose of antibiotics. The humanistic side, however, whether called "art" or not, is only dispensed by a human practitioner. If we fail to do this very thing, we fail to be physicians.

One type of problem in the emergency department that often turns out to be interesting is the type that checks in with a chief complaint of "talk to the doctor." Another form of this is the "personal" or "personal problem" complaint. These are usually of such a private nature, often sexual in origin, that the patient doesn't want to share the problem with the nursing staff and declines any further elaboration as to the true description of what's gone wrong. This event occurred on a Saturday night, near 10:00 p.m. or 11:00 p.m., just as things in the ED were going full swing. A thirty-something man was brought to the exam area, with the complaint of "talk to doctor." I picked up the chart and entered the room with my nicest "How can I help you?" voice. I saw no obvious blood, but he looked a little pale and was sitting on one of the side chairs in the exam room rather than on the exam table.

He said quietly and simply, "Doc, I broke my dick."

I looked at him carefully, without even the crack of a smile, and said, "Do you mean you've injured your penis?"

Now penis injuries are not all that uncommon. I mean, I've seen objects caught inside the urethra, objects trapped around the penis shaft, and injuries to the glans (tip) or foreskin, some of which are enumerated elsewhere in this series of tales. However, despite the teenage vernacular, referring to an erection as a *bone* or *boner*, I knew that erections are caused by a vascular tube of tissue that, when the central nervous system causes a muscular valve to close, fills with blood, and the engorgement produces the firmly rigid shaft that allows sexual intercourse. This erectile sac, actually a pair of them, one on either side of the urethra, lay along the length of the penis, underneath the skin, and travel the length of the member, whether hard or soft. Erections are *not* caused by a bone in the penis.

He nodded his head. "Yes," he said, "it's broken." I asked him to change into a gown, and I went out for a moment.

The nurse found me in the hallway and said, "Do you need some help?"

"No," I said, "I think that I've got this one covered." I reentered the room to find him, still apprehensive, sitting on the edge of the exam bed, with his bare feet dangling, knees apart. I pulled out the extension of the exam table and let him lie back. I draped his legs with a sheet and drew up the gown. He was right. It was broken. The shaft was purple, swollen around the middle, and bent at an awkward angle to the right from the midportion of the shaft. I gently examined the penis, checked the glans for blood, checked for injury at the base of the penis and the testes, and checked for pain in the inguinal regions adjacent to the genitals.

"What happened?" I asked.

"Well, I was on a date, and…you know, we were having sex, and I slipped out, and you know, I tried to reenter, and it wouldn't go, and I felt a *pop* and felt the pain, and it…broke. I mean it was loud enough that you could hear it."

I said that I'd need to get a consult with a urologist so that he (the patient) could have a surgical repair of the tissues that had torn.

He asked, "Don't we need to get an x-ray or something before surgery?" I quickly taught him the relevant anatomy. I asked when he'd last eaten, asked about allergies, past history, and so forth.

It turned out he was divorced for a year or so and had recently reentered the dating scene and was on a date while his mother was watching his two boys at home. Things had been working out very well for the date until the injury. As if the injury wasn't enough embarrassment, I observed the very painful phone call that he then made to his mother, telling her that he was not going to be home that night to pick up the boys, that he was at the hospital emergency room for a "minor problem," and that he would be having a minor surgery right away.

The portion of the conversation from the hospital room was "No, Mom, I'm not telling you why. I won't be home to pick up the boys. No, it's just a minor procedure. No, I don't want you to come to the hospital. No, Mom, don't come to the hospital. No, I'll pick up the boys tomorrow morning. No, Mom, don't come over to the hospital…"

Poor guy, I thought. That was turning out to be an expensive date. The story developed an even funnier side the following shift when the urologist stopped by the emergency department. I asked how the case had gone as he pulled an x-ray from an envelope. The x-ray, obviously contrived, showed the shadow of the male genitalia, with a superimposed chicken leg bone, carefully broken in the middle, exactly overlying the shadow of the penis.

"See?" he said, "there is a bone in there."

Laws of God, Laws of Man

On holiday weekends, the emergency department can get very busy. Staffing is always increased on such days, in anticipation of increased patient loads. Most times, however, it is still busy, and the staff will work long stretches without taking breaks for lunch or rest.

One such holiday, a Memorial Day weekend, I was on duty in the ED for the day shift. The day was busy, which, gratefully, made it go by quickly. After I finished my patients and dictated my charts, the department was still under siege by a larger-than-average number of patients. As I left the department, I saw several of the nurses that had been working straight through since their shift changed hours earlier. Doctors and nurses usually change shifts at different times and on different schedules, so as to maintain some continuity in the care of the patients. Grateful to be going home, I was looking forward to putting the top down on my Chrysler LeBaron convertible and feeling the wind blow through my thinning hair, happy to have someone else responsible for the patient flow. That was the nice thing about emergency medicine. Someone could take over for you, and you could turn the department over seamlessly, without any remorse or regret at the end of a shift. It became someone else's workload, and you didn't have to carry a pager or a phone or be on call. As I made a turn onto the street just outside the hospital parking lot, I was relishing in my freedom when I was struck with compassion for my coworkers back in the ED. I saw all the cars in the parking lot and knew that it might be hours yet, before there was a letup in new patients. On weekends and holidays, the emergency department was often the only medical facility open to assist members of a community with unplanned illness and injuries. I thought it would be nice if I took a few minutes before going home to stop by a local grocery to purchase some snacks and treats for the staff I'd just left behind. I often brought treats to the department, both for myself and as a bribe for the nursing staff. I didn't know what it was, they just seemed to look out for you and your patients a little better with chocolate in their breath.

I detoured down a street that I seldom travel, thinking over in my mind about what might be good to purchase to take back as a treat. I was absent-mindedly driving down the street, with visions of bags of red licorice, peanut M&Ms, ready-sliced fruit, and other favorite nurse bribes when I noticed two guys standing in the street up ahead. There was a pair of policeman, standing in my lane, immediately next to a parked patrol cruiser and pointing a radar gun at my vehicle. I realized that I didn't even know what the posted speed limit was on that street. As I got closer, the officer furthest from the patrol car motioned for me to pull over and stop. I recognized both of the officers from their visits earlier in the day with victims of some automobile accidents and other events, and they recognized me. They both walked up to the driver's side of my vehicle with broad grins.

"Do you know how fast you were going, Dr. Davis?"

"No," I said, "I wasn't paying much attention to the speedometer." I quickly thought that things might go better for me if I shared my selfless altruistic mission of mercy. "I was just on my way home and decided to swing by the supermarket to get some treats to take back to my poor, beleaguered coworkers in the emergency department, who have been working nonstop all day," and waited for their reply. Here I was, a hardworking emergency room doctor who had spent the day in the service of others. Surely, they'd understand my eagerness to accomplish my last altruistic task of the day and overlook absent-mindedness about the posted speed limit. I was hoping for a little selective enforcement. One of the officers was staring into the back seat of my car. *Uh-oh,* I thought. *What interested him there? Did I have something unexpected in my back seat?* I'm not prone to having contraband in my vehicle, and the worst that was usually there was an empty wrapper of something that I'd hurriedly eaten on the way to or from something. What had caught his attention? He leaned over and picked something out of my back seat. I turned around to see what it was. He was holding a zipped-up case that held my scriptures. I'd tossed them into the back seat last week after church. He smiled ear-to-ear, very proud of his next question.

"Dr. Davis," he said very piously, "how are you ever going to obey the laws of God when you can't even obey the laws of man?" as he tossed the book back in my car, he and his partner were doubled over in laughter.

"Drive slowly to the store and home," he warned. As I pulled away, I noticed in the rearview mirror that both of them were still standing in the street, laughing very, very loudly. I also noticed that my face was very, very red. Still to this day, several years later, that officer would remind me of my little criminal act and ask if I'd ever been able to come up with an answer for his question.

Fingerprint on Eye (Repeat)

Night shifts can be difficult for many reasons. Even during a series of back-to-back nights, you really never acclimate to being up all night, so you're thinking and diagnostic skills are always a little less than spectacular. Patients don't usually like to come to the emergency room at night, either, so they tend to stay home until things get really, really bad, or until they have lost all patience with whatever problem or pain is bugging them. This meeting between doctor and patient generally begins with an unknown medical problem. In these middle-of-the-night situations, it becomes a matter of patience, just being a good detective and even taking on some of the characteristics of Sherlock Holmes by looking at the whole patient in context and hunting down very small and seemingly insignificant clues. One such situation occurred in the early morning hours of one of my night shifts. A young mother brought in two boys. One child, the actual patient, was about three, and the other appeared to be about five. Her complaint upon arrival to the emergency department was that the younger boy "wouldn't stop crying.". She was carrying the younger child on her shoulder, and he, indeed, would not stop crying. Some children cry a lot in the emergency department when confronted by the white-coated doctor. This child, however, was really, really screaming. His fists were clenched. His eyes were closed, and he was relentless in his rather shrieking. His older brother seemed to be unaffected by it all and simply walked quietly to the room trailing his mother. I talked to the mother and was unable to get any other information about what might be causing the child to cry. She denied the child having any fever, chills, or other signs of illness. She was not aware of any recent injury, but agreed that the child, who slept in bunk beds with his older brother above him, might have fallen on his arm "or something." He had not had any similar episodes in the past. He took no medications and really had no significant past history. The kids were clean and well-dressed, even for two in the morning. I got no visual clues about possible injury or abuse, and the boys certainly didn't look neglected in any way.

I tried to approach him in an orderly fashion starting with his head and proceeding downward. One of the more common causes of pain in children is earache, so I, of course, checked both his ears, but I also checked for sore throat, nasal congestion, swollen lymph glands, and other signs of illness around the head or neck. I listened carefully to his lungs and heart and checked his tummy and found him normal in all respects. He didn't seem to have any pain movements of his arms or legs and had no difficulty moving his neck, back, or spine. I felt comfortable ruling out meningitis and earache. He didn't have a fever, and I couldn't find any other signs of illness. I carefully checked his hands, fingers, toes, and the rest of his extremities to see if he had any bruising or other signs of trauma. This kid was normal in every respect except that he kept screaming. After looking them over carefully from head to toe, I again talked with the mother to see if I could find any other history, and there was none. I even asked the brother if he'd seen the child fall or suffer any other injury, and he shook his head "no". I had no choice but to go over him from head to toe once again. This was the strangest case I'd had in some time because he had absolutely no physical findings. Despite this, he continued to scream at the top of his lungs, clinging to his mother's shoulder. I consulted with the nurse to see if she had seen any abnormalities and was just getting ready to get some laboratory tests to help me with the diagnosis when it suddenly occurred to me that the child had not once stopped screaming, nor had he once opened his eyes. When I examined his eyes, I had to pry them open, but after my exam, he immediately clenched them shut again. This was unusual because usually children would try to look around to determine their surroundings, and this child didn't. I confirmed this finding by prying open his eyes again and watched him quickly clenched them back closed. There wasn't any speck of dust or foreign material in his eyes that I could see, but he certainly didn't like them open. I went to the refrigerator and got some anesthetic drops for the eye and carefully placed them into the child's eyes. A few seconds later, the child, opened his eyes, and looked around. This was the first time he had stopped crying since before entering the emergency department. I then placed some coloring agent into the eyes and found my answer. There, on the surface of his left cornea was a small fingerprint. Just about the size of his brother's fingers. I turned to the brother, looked him squarely in the eye, and said "Did you poke your brother in the eye?"

He looked at me very sheepishly and nodded "yes".

His mother was relieved to find that she would only have to use some eye drops overnight for his "eye print" and that his eye would feel better by morning. I was relieved to have solved a deep, deep mystery.

Broken Thermometer

As I've mentioned, a large portion of emergency medicine occurs in the investigation of chief complaints. Sometimes this requires true ingenuity, but so can the resulting treatment procedures, which oftentimes rise to the level of MacGyver.

One such case involved the mother who rushed her child into the emergency department with the complaint that she had a sick child and had been taking the child's temperature with a rectal thermometer when the child had twisted, causing the thermometer to break off inside the child's rectum. A quick exam showed that there was no bleeding present, but the mother did have in her hand half of the offending thermometer with a sharp, flap-shaped edge at its distal end. The next step of evaluation of this potentially serious injury was to obtain an x-ray both in the AP and lateral directions, looking for the glass and mercury of the thermometer. Upon return of the child from x-ray and viewing the pictures, I said, "I found it. There it is," seeing about an inch and a half long shadow from a glass-thermometer-shaped object, complete with the expanded bulb at the distal end and present about two inches into the rectum. Again, I noticed no bleeding or blood on the diaper. As I was thinking through the management of this problem, I thought I really needed an endoscope that would allow me to look into the rectal area and grasp the thermometer and retrieve it. From the x-ray, I could tell that a flap of glass projected from the broken remnant of that piece of the thermometer and appeared to be oriented such that it was embedding itself into the wall of the sigmoid colon. I was inspired by a trick I had learned elsewhere in medicine. Using a small 7 mL glass test tube, inserting it into the rectal opening after removing the stopper, I could use it as a very small scope and examine the rectal mucosa. Using plenty of lubrication, the child tolerated this very well, and after advancing the inverted tube two inches into the rectal area, I was rewarded by the broken-off glass thermometer segment dropping into the hollow cavity of the inverted test tube with a loud clunk. The test tube had both served to allow entry into the child's rectum as well as to stretch the outer mucosa allowing the sharp tip of the thermometer fragment to disengage from the mucosal wall and drop into the waiting receptacle. This was not followed by any bleeding. For a while there, I was known as MacGyver around the emergency department because of the success of this maneuver. It resulted in the retrieval of the glass fragment of the thermometer without any further trauma to the child's rectum and was actually a painless procedure. I thought about filing this away under "useful tips," but I really didn't know when I would use it again.

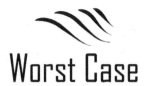

Worst Case

During the fifteen-plus years that I worked as a full-time emergency physician, I was often asked, "So what is the worst case you've ever seen?" So this is a very interesting question, and the answer is, "It depends." The truth is, it depends on what you consider the worst case. Now in this book, I've described several cases that had multiple injured victims, and those certainly meet qualifications of *worst case* just based on the presence of suffering by humanity. What people usually mean, however, is what is the "most gruesome case" that you can think of off the top of your head. This is because people love to slow down at the scene of an accident, love to imagine an injured person in the back of an ambulance, and love to pick the brain of a practicing ER doctor in case there's some good blood and gore to be shared. I'll try not to disappoint.

One such case that would qualify as a *worst case* would be a situation that presented one weekend while I was moonlighting in the emergency room of the town of Price, Utah. Now this community is located in the mining area within the center part of the state.

While providing care there, I participated in the care of victims of mining accidents, including cave-ins, severe mechanical trauma such as crush injuries, broken bones, lacerations, etc., as well as the usual rural farm accidents, vehicular trauma, and other things that kept me very busy while performing those shifts. One case, however, stands out in my mind as, while being unrelated to any of the aforementioned sources of disease or injury, it was related to the recreational activities associated with this part of the state and involved a school bus that had been converted by the family into a weekend camper. My initial contact with his case came by notification via ambulance radio that the local EMTs were responding along with the local fire department, to a possible camper fire. As word continued to arrive from the scene, located about twenty minutes away from Price, we were informed that while the camper had been mostly consumed by the fire, the family was thought to be safely accounted for. About forty-five minutes later, I was notified of the arrival of an ambulance at the doorway of the hospital and the presence of two EMTs/firemen who had a singularly unique problem. In the course of searching through the fire, they became aware that an infant child of this family was unaccounted for, and they were sent to search through the burned remains of the camper in an attempt to locate the possible whereabouts of this small infant. I really had nothing more than that, including no confirmation of the possible tragedy because members of the family who remained at the campsite were not clear with the responding fireman as to whether or not the child was taken to safety from the campsite or whether the child had indeed suffered exposure to the burning bus.

The firemen had a simple question. "We've brought something in. We need to know whether it is a baby or not."

Of course, I steeled myself to prepare for what I might discover. What they brought had the appearance of what could've been a mattress or other debris but had no discernible shape or identifiable origin. The material was wrapped in a sheet that had been salvaged from the ambulance at the scene of the fire. I brought the bundle into the emergency department, placed it by the sink, and began to unwrap it. Now I have a pretty strong stomach, but I was unprepared by the discovery of the charred remains of a small infant who had been severely burned almost beyond recognition. My immediate reaction was to turn to the sink in uncontrolled emesis. Over the course of my service in the emergency department, I only had very few cases that affected me in that manner. I mentioned the open-heart-surgery case that caused me to become lightheaded and dizzy. This was also the case the first time I witnessed electroconvulsive therapy in the psych unit, but I was, for the most part, unaffected by the sights and smells of emergency medicine, including ruptured appendices, surgery on bowel obstructions, and various presentations of pus and other infected fluids. This extremely sad case therefore topped my list, as it likely should.

Another candidate for the *worst case* had to be a young man who presented to my emergency department late one Friday at about 1 o'clock in the morning. This case came to the emergency department with about six- or seven-minute notice having been the result of a quick *scoop and run* by the community paramedics. They had responded to the victim's home where they found a young man in his late teens who suffered from a self-inflicted gunshot wound to the face. They reported that this was result of a gun cleaning accident and did not give a history of any suicidal ideation or intent. The end result was that the patient had effectively removed most of his lower jaw, suffered injury to his upper jaw, and a large portion of the skin of his face and one eye. Now I must mention that I had actually seen this type of injury once previously during my Tremonton practice years from a similar mechanism. This prior experience allowed me to act rapidly to assess and implement a treatment plan.

My first response was to begin stabilization of the patient by starting a large-bore IV, sending blood to be crossmatched and typed, and asking for type O negative blood from the laboratory. Fortunately, I had two good nurses on duty that night for assistance. I sent one of them to page for the on-call anesthesia doctor to come to the ED to help me in obtaining and stabilizing the patient's airway. He was moving air pretty well without assistance, but I readily saw that there was no way that he would easily be able to continually protect his airway due to the jaw injury. There was just too much blood and loose tissue present to apply a mask and not enough recognizable, uninjured anatomy to be certain of tube placement. I started a large subclavian line and awaited the arrival of the anesthesiologist. Within just a few minutes, the anesthesiologist appeared in the doorway of the patient's room and stopped and stared with a vacant look at the presenting scene. He stood there, literally with open mouth, and didn't say a word. I turned to him with urgency in my eyes and said, "You going to help me with this airway, aren't you?" He didn't respond but just continued to stare, apparently paralyzed by the shocking scene before him. I asked him two more times if he could assist me, and he never did respond. I finally reached around him in the doorway, pulled the curtain closed to block his view, and proceeded to obtain the placement of an ET tube through the injured oral cavity. This procedure successfully resulted in the obtaining of a stable airway that continued to serve through the remainder of the resuscitation. The air ambulance was called, responded with their ETA, and we continued to prepare the patient for transfer. By the time the air ambulance arrived, the patient had available transfusible blood, with all of his laboratory tests completed, a visit by his parents, and other housekeeping matters taken care of. The placement of a urinary catheter, after the arrival of the Life Flight helicopter, the patient was hot loaded for transport, and the flight team gave instructions to the parents as to the future location of their son. Although this case went very smoothly, in no small part due to my prior experience with this type of case, it was not the type of case that I ever wanted to see very often. I saw the patient a few times in the ensuing years after he had undergone multiple maxillofacial repair surgeries, and I'm happy to report a good outcome with a functioning lower jaw, the ability to eat, breathe effectively, and even speak in a somewhat garbled voice.

To this day, I'm not certain what froze the anesthesiologist in the doorway except for the gruesome initial surprise that greeted him that night. I often wonder if I couldn't have done more to prepare him for that scene.

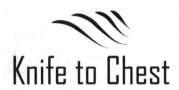

Knife to Chest

Another interesting case was the direct result of living in a college town with young adults. One Saturday night in the early evening, paramedics brought a twenty-year-old to the emergency department with a knife sticking out of his chest. His history, as they related it, was that the patient was enjoying a Saturday evening dinner with his girlfriend. The patient became upset at some element of their conversation, reached up onto the table, grasped a steak knife, and thrust it into his own chest. This was in an attempt to take his own life. The paramedics had restrained the patient from further attempts at self-injury for their transport. There in the patient's chest stood an upright knife that had obviously penetrated its full length into the chest cavity and with each heartbeat bobbing back and forth in time with the beating heart. After securing a large-bore IV, sending blood for typing crossmatch, listening to the lungs, and verifying adequate ventilation, I tried to find more about the patient.

He was, indeed, a young man on a date with his girlfriend, but she had broken off their date prior to the incident. My training taught me not to attempt to remove an embedded foreign body in the chest or any other location due to the probability of increased risk of bleeding or trauma to the lung or clearly to the adjacent beating heart. The patient had several sets of vital signs by the time of arrival in the emergency department and was clearly stable to a degree. Because of the obvious need for thoracic surgery exploration, I immediately placed a call to summon Life Flight and sent the appropriate staff to prepare the landing site. We again obtained several units of crossmatch blood, which we intended to send along with the Life Flight team. He also had a Foley catheter placed and was constantly monitored for blood oxygenation because of the chest injury. Throughout his stay, he experienced no shortness of breath but did have chest pain from the obvious source. Also throughout his stay, each passing heartbeat continued to cause the knife to deflect from its embedded position in a regular pattern, indicating close proximity to the beating heart. A chest x-ray was obtained, which did not clearly define the pathway of penetration. Because his breathing remained stable, he did not require the immediate replacement of the chest tube, but we carefully watched for the development of a pneumothorax or other respiratory decompensation.

I was faced with the challenge of safely transporting this patient the distance of approximately one hundred miles in the air ambulance with a knife sticking out of his chest. I thought in my mind several times about how I could support that knife, given its throbbing movements and protruding position with respect to the chest wall. I settled on the novel idea of stabilizing the knife handle with a cardboard tube from a roll of paper towels by cutting the edge of the tube into a *T* shape, taping it to the chest wall without restricting the knife movement or further injuring the chest, and prepared for the arrival of Life Flight. When the blood was available and Life Flight had arrived, I gave them the rundown on the patient's history thus far and the stability of his condition. We carefully transferred the patient to a rolling cart and brought him to the helicopter landing site outside of the emergency department. I helped the Life Flight crew transfer him carefully into the aircraft, very careful not to bump the protruding knife. With the patient stabilized in this manner, they were successful in transporting him all the way to the waiting thoracic surgeon at the Salt Lake City area hospital. I later received an envelope in the mail from Life Flight that contained several photographs of my jury-rigged or MacGyvered external chest-wall-stabilization device because they were so impressed with the successful implementation of that device. I couldn't help but think that despite being a simple, "dumb country doctor," I had configured an emergency device that protected the patient's chest wall during the transport journey.

"Even a blind sow gets an acorn every so often" was an adage that came to mind from my Iowa farm days.

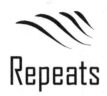

Repeats

One of the questions that I'm often asked is "What is the stupidest thing you've ever seen?" Over the years, I've had a lot of time to think about this question, and my answer has become, "No, it's not the stupidest thing I've ever seen. It's the unluckiest thing I've ever seen. However, if you do it again, it will be the stupidest thing I've ever seen!"

An exemplary case of this was on one working day when the patient entered the emergency department with a chief complaint of *lacerated leg*. The history was the patient had cut his leg with a chainsaw while working at a construction site a few blocks from the hospital. The chainsaw blade had torn through the patient's blue jeans and had lacerated through the skin and underlying muscle. The vital structures underneath were for the most part uninjured, and there was no serious bleeding. The wound however was contaminated by wood chips, shredded blue jeans, and devitalized muscle. Just the kind of case I liked! Following the numbing of the skin with local anesthetic, I irrigated the wound with sterile saline and removed all the particles of wood, shreds of denim, and devitalized tissue.

The wound edges closed very well despite the injury to the muscle and the bulk of the patient's muscular thigh. Likewise, the skin closed over the wound, with the fascia first and then skin sutures. With this complete, I proceeded to instruct the patient in aftercare. I was concerned that due to the depth of the laceration, the patient might have subsequent bleeding from the injured muscle edges. I gave him specific instructions that included going home to rest, not returning to work, keeping the leg elevated, and watching carefully for redness or infection with further instructions to return should any sign of complication develop. The patient received these instructions both verbally and in writing and agreed to return for suture removal in about ten to fourteen days.

The patient was able to walk without a limp despite the muscular injury. As he headed out the door, I said, "Now don't go back to work."

To which, he replied, "I have to go tell my boss I won't be able to come back, but otherwise, I'll go home."

A few minutes later, I saw the patient walk back around the doorway of the emergency department and initially thought, *Well, he's forgotten his wallet or something and is returning to get it.* No, the patient had in that short time span returned to his job site, returned to the chainsaw, picked it up, and started cutting wood once again, and in his weakened state, he had let the saw slip, cutting off his large toe on the same leg previously injured. There you go, very unlucky, indeed! Or was it dumb?

Sometimes in emergency medicine, it's hard to differentiate between plain *bad luck* and pure Darwinian at its finest. I've gotten a lot of smiles and entertainment value over trying to differentiate between the two. When I see you as a patient, however, I'm very likely to give you the benefit of the doubt. At least the first time.

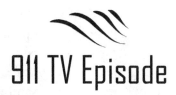

911 TV Episode

One winter day, I believe it was a Saturday, I received an ambulance call stating that we had an inbound ambulance from the Bear Lake area with a near-drowning victim on board. While drownings are not rare at Bear Lake, this one was quite unusual because of the time of the year—midwinter. The story received from the ambulance was this was one of our deputy sheriffs, a member of the local underwater search and rescue team, who was doing some practice dives through the ice at Bear Lake. His group consisted of his wife, who was his surface tender, and a dive buddy would also be under the ice at the time of the accident. This was an interesting story as I learned that the pair of divers had cut a hole in the ice a short ways offshore, prepared their equipment, then under close watch by the patient's wife had entered the cold waters of Bear Lake through ice. Both divers were tethered to a guide rope that was tended by the wife, the third member of the party. The patient had apparently entered the water, started his practice dive by swimming away from the opening in the ice, but the two divers became separated; at which time, the dive buddy turned around and followed his rope back to the ice opening and slowly popped up on the surface and asked the dive tender where her husband was. This caused some alarm on the part of the tender, and she immediately tugged on the rope and received no reassuring tug in reply. She reported that after just a few tugs on the rope, the body of her husband, not moving nor apparently breathing, was found in the ice a couple of feet from the center of the opening. The buddy diver, also a deputy sheriff, and the wife performed CPR on the victim, which resulted in the spontaneous return of respirations and awakening from being unconscious. They immediately called the ambulance that responded and brought the patient, now revived, to the emergency department to be checked for signs and symptoms of near drowning. I saw the patient after he was fully revived and carefully examined him for signs of water aspiration and any other ill effects from his near-death experience. Because Bear Lake is approximately thirty-five minutes away by ambulance, he was fully revived coherent and able to cooperate with his examination. It turned out that he had no long-term ill effects, no sign of freshwater drowning including water intoxication, and didn't even have a residual cough. After observing him in the emergency department for a safe period, he was released into the care of his wife.

Sometime later, several months after the initial event, I received a phone call from the patient who said that he had reported the event to the producers of the TV show called *Rescue 911* and that they had accepted this event for future filming for one of their TV episodes. They planned to come to the Logan area to interview the physician and staff who provided the care on the day of the event, as well as interview the victim, his wife, and dive buddy. They planned to recreate the event for TV as one of their episodes of the weekly television program.

The weekly TV show was hosted by William Shatner, one of my favorite TV personalities, and I looked forward to the opportunity of perhaps making his acquaintance. On the day scheduled for the arrival of the television crew, I was sorry to learn that Mr. Shatner would not be attending, but I would meet with one of the two cameramen and the producer of the episode in question. They came to the ED on my day off and met with me as scheduled. Now this was again midwinter the following year, and I had grown out a full beard in celebration of the cold weather and no-shave November. It was with this appearance that I met with the producer and cameramen. The producer was new to Utah, it being his first trip from the coast, and the first question he asked me was "Are you a Mormon? And how many wives do you have?" I assured him that I only had a single spouse, and we laughed and joked about a few of the other differences between Utah and the rest of the world at the West Coast.

He then proceeded to set up the cameras and question me about the events of that day, one year previous that resulted in the near-drowning experience. I described the events of that day, including the benefits of the CPR provided by the spouse, the rapid transport of the near-drowning victim, and the fortuitous coincidence that resulted in the rapid retrieval of the victim. Apparently, soon after entering the water, the victim had become entangled in the tender ropes that resulted in his body being pulled back to the opening in the ice by his dive buddy as the dive buddy swam back to the opening. This meant that the wife found the floating victim after just a couple of short tugs on the tender rope and likely shortened his exposure time under the water and helped to ensure his successful resuscitation. Apparently, upon entry into the water, the patient's dive air regulator had become supercooled by the frosty air at the altitude of the dive, and this supercooled air had caused the victim's regulator to freeze, which stopped supplying his breathing air. His dive buddy had recognized the loss of air pressure, but the victim apparently had run out of air and had passed out, unconscious, while being dragged back to the opening in the ice. At any rate, it was a rapid and successful resuscitation performed by his quick-thinking spouse, who had been trained in CPR and had successfully resuscitated him.

After hearing my recitation of the story, the director asked me, "So did she save his life?"

I was proud of her successful efforts, proud to be a part of the story, and proud of my community. I thought very quickly about the producer's original comment and, as a joke, looked straight at the camera and said, "Yes, I do think she saved his life. I don't know if many of my wives would've done that." He and I immediately burst into laughter, but resuming his director's role, he yelled, "Cut! Wait, what is that you said?"

We had a good laugh and then shot the retake where I just said in all seriousness, "Yes, she certainly did save his life."

It is perhaps of interest that later that day, as the film crew moved to a local freshwater reservoir in order to recreate the on-ice and underwater circumstances that had caused the near drowning, the regulators of the two cameramen had experienced similar subzero temperatures preparatory to the dive, and so during the actual dive recreation, the two regulators had both frozen, causing the underwater photographers to run out of air and struggle to the surface of the ice before losing consciousness. I guess this was an example of true reality TV. Another postscript was that when it came time to air the actual episode recreation, I was there on Tuesday evening, glued to the TV, to see my chance at national stardom come to life. I carefully watched the episode segment dealing with my patient and learned that they had edited out all my footage and concentrated only on the events that occurred up at Bear Lake. Nonetheless, it was a good teaching episode for the benefits of knowing CPR and explaining the risks of wintertime ice diving.

Miscarriage Answer to Blessing

One night, I experienced a particularly busy weekend shift and was looking forward expectantly, to closing out and going home. My replacement had already arrived, but because I had fallen a little behind, I decided to finish up by helping see the patients, already in the department, to help my replacement catch up. It was under these circumstances that I went in to see my final patient of the evening, a young twentyish female who was accompanied by an older woman, who introduced herself as the patient's mother. The patient's chief complaint was *vaginal bleeding*. The patient was noticeably quiet, and I believed this to be due to some discomfort that she was probably experiencing and proceeded to take her history. She was early in her second trimester, had noticed some active spotting/bleeding, and had come to the ER for evaluation. This was her first pregnancy, and so I assumed that she was frightened, in addition to being uncomfortable, and talked with her about the process that we would go through toward confirming the viability of the pregnancy, her Rh-factor status, and other details for her safety and care. Her mother sat quietly while I interviewed the patient, but I could tell that the mother wanted to talk with me to give me some additional history. After ordering the blood work and the sonogram, I went to my desk and began dictating the remainder of my charts from the previous busy shift.

Out of the corner of my eye, I saw the mother of the patient in the nurses' station, apparently looking for assistance. I stopped dictating and asked if I could help her.

She said, "I want to tell you about my daughter." This lady related to me some additional information, including several things that helped my understanding as to why the patient was so quiet when I was questioning her. She told me that the young woman was married, but that her husband had left her about ten days earlier, saying that he did not any longer want to be married to her and was abandoning his wife and child to move out of the home. The young mother-to-be was reportedly quite sad over the breakup of her marriage and had become very depressed as a result. This, she hoped, would help me understand a little bit more about her daughter's mood in the face of profound depression. I thanked her for the additional information and returned to my charting. Several minutes later, the daughter returned from ultrasound, and I was happy to share with her the results.

The exam showed a viable fetus around sixteen weeks gestation with the fetus showing good activity, strong heartbeat, and normal location of the placenta. I reviewed with her the blood type and Rh, as well as her lack of anemia and overall good health. I asked her if she had a chance to see her baby during the ultrasound study. She said that she had not been able to see the screen from her position on the mobile cart because the screen was directed at the ultrasound tech and beyond her visibility. My own daughter had recently experienced a full miscarriage during a pregnancy, so I knew how frightening this could be to an expectant mother. I don't know why, but something told me to take the time to use the departmental ultrasound to go to the patient's bedside and repeat the ultrasound for the patient's benefit so that she could see an image of her unborn child. Now remember, I was done with my shift, and this was all being done during time that I normally would have been driving home to my family. I pulled the ultrasound machine from its storage spot, applied gel to the patient's round abdomen, and pressed the buttons on the machine to start the image and began scanning the pelvis for the pregnancy. I easily found the image of the unborn baby. It was free-floating like a tiny little spaceman within the amniotic fluid. It was very physically active moving his arms and legs in the fluid. The heartbeat was regular, and I could actually see the valves opening and closing in the chest. I showed the mother the heartbeat, showed the arms and legs, but couldn't, at that time, determine the future gender. Right at that moment, the child, who was active in kicking, chose to raise his arm and produce a sort of a wave to the mother, clearly visible on the screen.

I said, "Oh look, your baby is waving at you." The mother gasped but didn't say anything as the patient silently looked on. We finished the scanning with more reassurance that the pregnancy was indeed viable and healthy, and there was not a dangerous source found for the spotting. I finished instructing her on the aftercare for the visit, including things to watch for, how soon to follow up with her primary care doctor, and continue her prenatal care. I thanked her for the experience, still feeling just a little emotional for what she was going through but relieved that I could be reassuring at this point in time of a good chance of a successful outcome.

I was back to dictating my final chart when the patient's mother approached my workspace and said, "Could I talk with you?"

I said, "Certainly, what can I help you with?"

The patient's mother said, "Do you realize that you are an answer to exactly what she needed tonight?"

I said, "How so?"

The grandmother-to-be related that the patient had experienced reservations about continuing with the pregnancy but had not wanted to terminate the pregnancy due to her religious beliefs. This left her with a dilemma of whether or not to become a single mother, and so she had sought help from her spiritual advisers, which had resulted in the calling of two elders from her church to come to her home and offer her a priesthood blessing for spiritual comfort and assistance. During the blessing, the elders had pronounced their hope that the patient would resolve her feelings of indifference toward this pregnancy, that the threatened miscarriage situation would resolve safely, and that the patient would not experience long-term adversity as a result. Additionally, they went further to express their feeling that the patient would return to a state of well-being and would come to develop a healthy relationship with the future child. She further related that, in her opinion, my demonstration with the ultrasound was the answer to the prayers of her daughter because she had indeed witnessed events that had furthered her development of a relationship with the unborn child.

Since that night, I reflected on that event on many occasions. It remained very close to my heart and generated many deep emotions. I was grateful to have had the opportunity to participate in the care of this patient and the reassurance of the patient and her mother. I really don't know whether my actions constituted a true "answer to a prayer" or the fulfillment of a blessing. Nonetheless, I believe it was one of those experiences that I have had over the course of my career where I have been able to touch the life of one of my patients in a way that was uplifting and spiritually relevant to them while I met their needs. This is one of the benefits of having a front-row seat and being prepared at all times to experience sudden intimacy.

The Perfect Marriage

One of the stories that I learned early on in my career and liked to relate in later situations was something I witnessed regarding a perfect marriage. It was late on a weekend night when an elderly couple checked into the emergency department for problem complaint being experienced by the husband. The presentation wasn't so important as the lesson I learned about what constitutes a perfect marriage. The husband was dressed in his best suit of clothes, which was often the case with elderly gentleman in our area who are coming to the doctor because they always wore their best clothing. Likewise his wife, who accompanied him on this visit, was wearing a blue dress that had probably seen more of the insides of churches than I had. This nice-looking elderly couple was brought into the emergency department, placed in a room, and the husband, the one with the concern, was given a gown to wear. I entered his room, took a quick history, and immediately saw that I was going to need to order some laboratory evaluation to help sort out his concerns. The emergency department oftentimes was quiet at that early hour with no other patients around, and I was in the habit, if all my charting was caught up, of spending the time at the patient's bedside getting to know a little bit about them and had, as a result of this frequent activity, learned a lot of the local history and experiences of its elderly members.

I was done with my physical evaluation and was awaiting the return of laboratory tests, so I pulled up a chair next to the patient's bedside and started asking him questions about his life. His wife was seated in a side chair next to him and was hunched forward, leaning on her cane. She listened intently as I asked questions about his life.

He was in his mideighties and had seen and experienced many things that I, of course, had not.

As was the usual case, I asked an open-ended question, "In your eighty-some years, what's the most memorable thing you can remember?" He was a little hard of hearing and asked for the question to be repeated, and I believed that his wife repeated the question as well.

"In your eighty years, what's the most memorable thing that you can recall?" As he paused and pondered, he finally came up with an answer that I considered priceless.

He smiled at me and said, "Well, it was either when they landed a man on the moon or when I met my wife." He looked at her after the question in order to check her reaction to his response.

Without missing a beat, she stared at him intently, leaned forward on her cane for support, and said, raising her voice a little for emphasis, "Well, which was it?"

Without a moment's hesitation and patting the air in a dismissive fashion, he waved her off saying, "I'm thinking, I'm thinking." They both chuckled at this, seeming to have a good time. I realized that here they were in the wee hours of the morning with him experiencing some potentially significant health problems in their later years; they were best friends to each other. He was unashamed about challenging their relationship, and she was likewise willing to tease him back in return. This couple demonstrated to me that each of us ought to be able to, when life turns harsh, count on those closest to us for both physical and emotional support. This, to me, is a strong indicator of a healthy marriage. Later on, when I was dealing with students who often had questions about relationships and marriage, I used this case as an example of a perfect relationship of mutual support between two loving adults. The patient's test results returned, and I can't even remember the disposition of the case, whether he was admitted or discharged home, but I certainly remembered to this day that example of a loving and supportive marital relationship.

Number 1 Accidents That I Came Upon Where I Was the First Responder

One of the goals that I originally had in becoming an emergency physician was to put myself in a situation where I would always know or at least almost always know the correct treatment for the emergency. Most of my life had been involved in working within the confines of the emergency department itself and not venturing out into the realm of the first responder. There had been some situations, however, where my role had been that of a first responder and could see the medical emergency unfold before my eyes from the very onset. Fortunately, these were very rare, and I had the luxury of leaving the duties of the first responder to those special individuals who have the aptitude and demand for adrenaline that enables them to work day after day in the front lines of emergency services. As my career progressed, I became more actively involved in teaching these individuals starting with basic first aid and including EMTs, paramedics, medical students, and fellow physicians. I have to admit that I never considered myself to suffer from a need for adrenaline stimulation, and in fact, most of my first-response efforts were aimed at minimizing the apprehension that accompanies unplanned emergencies.

I was making a presentation to a group of assembled hospital administrators during an annual meeting gathering. This event occurred at a hotel about one hundred miles distant, and I was, therefore, required to stay overnight for the duration of the meeting. A scheduling conflict had developed with one of my boys in that his football team was playing a scheduled game at a high school field about forty miles further than the resort hotel. As a result of this, I planned to take my wife, speak at the conference, and after finishing the meetings, proceed the following day to the second location where the game would be played. The timing worked out well so that I could meet my obligation to my administrator, complete my drive, and attend the game where I would also function as the team physician.

Things were proceeding along the planned timeline, and I found myself driving along the back roads of rural Utah, taking a shortcut that included a beautiful canyon drive next to a bubbling stream, well-known for its trout fishing, which, at its end, would drop me directly near my planned destination. This area of Utah is somewhat mountainous, and because of the fall season, I was really enjoying the fall colors and other scenery. We were at a point well outside of the nearest community when a scene unveiled itself in front of me unexpectedly.

My wife and I came over a small hill with a beautiful vista laid out before us as we entered a wide straight stretch of road in a valley. Ahead of me, I saw a crossroad and witnessed a truck that was carrying raw timber toward a nearby sawmill. It was not slowing for the intersection, and I very quickly realized that his horn was also honking intermittently. I realized that he was warning oncoming traffic that his brakes had failed and that he was going to be unable to stop for cross traffic. There, about one hundred yards ahead of my current position, he slammed broadside into a passenger vehicle, spinning it around in a cloud of dust, where it came to rest in the middle of the road pointed to an awkward direction. His uncontrolled log truck proceeded to cross the road, go down into the ditch, and its momentum carried it about seventy yards further after the impact. Realizing that we were the only other vehicle visible at that point in time, I told my wife that I needed to stop to see if we could render some assistance.

The dust was still settling as I pulled to the side of the road, parked my car out of the travel path of the highway, turned on my emergency flashers, and ran to the impacted vehicle. The horn was still blaring loudly, and I noticed that there were two dazed passengers in the front seat of the vehicle. The driver, upon whose side the impact had occurred, was slumped forward, her hands resting and nonmoving across the steering column. There was obvious injury to her head and face, and I quickly determined that she was not breathing nor responsive to my verbalizations to her. Her passenger, also in the front seat, was drowsy but responsive and was very frightened.

Her first words to me were "I think my mother is dead." Almost immediately, I saw a second vehicle, coming from the opposite direction, pulled to a stop, with the driver exiting the vehicle.

A young woman approached hurriedly and said, "I am a nurse. Can I be of help?" The two of us confirmed the lack of responsiveness or breathing from the driver and then proceeded to concentrate our efforts on the passenger. I called out to my wife instructing her to call 911 and have the dispatcher respond an ambulance.

Although I was in an unfamiliar territory, I knew approximately my location and also knew that the nearest hospital was a small, rural facility in a community that I estimated to be about ten or twelve miles distant. I confirmed that my patient was breathing without pain or stridor, but had some neck pain despite her having been wearing her seatbelt. She was also complaining of some bruising on her forehead from the violent impact. At about this time, the driver of the runaway truck walked up to the accident scene having brought his truck to stop amid some trees and stood there in a state of shock, having witnessed the effects of his collision. Over the next several minutes, other travelers stopped, and I assigned bystanders to help direct traffic flow and used still others to position and hold the cervical collar and IV setup, which I retrieved from my first-aid kit that I always had packed in the back of my SUV. This particular day, I was fortunate to also be carrying my sideline kit, anticipating its use at the football game later that day. This meant that I had access to an extensive number of dressings that were clean and sterile.

My wife told me that it would be about twenty to thirty minutes duration before we could expect the arrival of the ambulance that had been dispatched by the volunteer fire service in that small community. I knew that in the next valley west, approximately thirty miles over the mountains, set the city of Salt Lake City. This included two major trauma centers and several smaller hospitals. Armed with this geographic knowledge, I made the decision to directly summon an air ambulance to the scene of this fatal accident. My hospital system often uses the air ambulance service for transfers and consultation, so I knew the telephone number quite well. I dialed the number directly on my cell phone and was connected to their dispatch. I told the responding dispatcher who I was and the circumstances of my situation. He agreed to dispatch the air ambulance in accordance with my directions to our location. He predicted the flight time would be about twelve to fourteen minutes, and I proceeded to assign individuals to canvas the area adjacent to the highway for any litter that might be picked up by the rotor wash and cause potential harm to the aircraft. At about this time, I finally saw the red-and-blue lights of an approaching highway patrol vehicle.

I quickly brought the responding officer up to speed with regards to the injuries, the presence of a fatality, and the risks due to the high-energy impact, and the presence of neck pain. I told him of the pending time of arrival of the air ambulance, and he gratefully acknowledged the work of the bystanders, the first responding nurse, and me. He also provided a blanket to hang up in the driver-side window to block passing traffic from seeing the deceased driver. During the next several minutes, while the nurse started the IV and covered the exposed wounds, we accomplished identifying the landing zone, marking it with flares, and completed the setup for the arrival of the air ambulance. The air ambulance arrived on schedule, received a quick report from myself and the nurse, and lifted off for the return trip to their hospital.

I talked with the responding trooper, letting him know of my desire to proceed on my way to the football game and noted that I could still make it before game time. I gave him my contact information, told him what I had seen with regards to the impact and collision, and pointed out the truck driver, who was still pretty quiet and very much in shock from the ordeal.

I realized that I had been the beneficiary of some excellent roadside help in the form of a nurse, the responding trooper, and all the bystanders. I also realized that I was fortunate to have had a well-equipped first-aid kit and my sideline bag attending with me that day. These additional events certainly helped make the outcome more positive. In addition to the cervical collar, I also had an IV start kit and bag of IV fluids in my sideline bag, and the nurse and I were able to accomplish the opening of an IV line prior to the arrival of the helicopter. Thus, saving several minutes at the scene, allowing a rapid turnaround and departure.

Gratefully, he allowed me to leave the scene and continue on my way to the game. It took me several minutes of travel before my adrenaline level allowed me to communicate my impressions to my wife. She had always been very stoic but not much of a first responder or prone to jump into emergencies unnecessarily. However, she did not lose control or become a liability in emergency settings. She simply didn't like doing those kinds of things if she didn't have to. We completed the remainder of the drive, located the high school site of the football game, and returned to my scheduled role as a sideline physician for the local high school football team. We were a little late for pregame warm-ups but were there for the kickoff and had a great story to tell!

Hike the Tetons

One of the advantages of an emergency medicine practice was the access to an increased amount of free time over my previous practice site. This allowed me to undertake more leisure activities, including family time, vacations, and coaching my children's activities. These activities would've been nearly impossible in my previous circumstances. Because we live in northern Utah, we have available numerous active outdoor recreation opportunities, national parks, hiking trails, lakes, rivers, as well as indoor recreation opportunities.

I had visited grand Teton National Park, first as a child and later as an adult, and had longed to find myself hiking the trails, backpack on my back, with everything I needed self-contained. To this end, I had purchased several pieces of new equipment at REI and had contacted Teton National Park during one of my visits there to get further information about obtaining the required permits for overnight stays. It was my nature to study situations like this thoroughly before embarking, and so armed with maps, information, personally obtained advice, and other essentials, I found myself with a planned trip in mid-July to that national park. My two boys were unquestionably on board with our plans, and two of my daughters were definitely not interested, preferring instead to spend their time in Jackson Hole Wyoming, shopping. My wife's idea of "roughing it" was to sleep with the hotel window open, so I knew she wouldn't be of much benefit on the trip. My middle daughter was a bit of a question mark. She was very "green" and would have likely enjoyed the trip and the hiking experience but would have been the only female on the trip and was therefore, unfortunately, excluded in preference to my son-in-law. She had often reminded me of that lost opportunity for her and frequently wondered if I was fair in the selection process.

I spent the months of January through June firming up plans, obtaining supplies, planning menus, weighing equipment, and various other related activities in preparation for the upcoming trip. We had backpacks and supplies purchased, packed, and taken for brief introductory hikes prior to departure. We drove by jeep to the visitor center at Teton National Park and checked in with the ranger station there to verify our permits. There would be four of us on this trip, and we planned to spend two nights and three days on the trails surrounding the Grand Teton Mountain. We would be fully self-contained using pump filters to provide clean water, eating mostly dehydrated dried food, and caring only the essential items of clothing and toiletries. Because we were carrying everything on our backs with no planned resupply source, we were traveling light.

The trailhead was located just across Jenny Lake in an area called Cascade Canyon. The initial couple of hundred yards was steep, and I was thinking that it might be too difficult when I found the trail leveling out, and we began what became a gentle climb around the southern view of the grand. We were nearly alone on the trail but were carefully watching for flowers and other notable scenery with one eye carefully watching for bears. We had discussed the current bear situation with the park rangers and found that there were no current significant threats. We still were planning on being very conscientious about camp hygiene, not leaving food lying around, and protecting our supplies by hanging them from a rope in a tree near our campsite.

After a couple of hours of walking, we noticed we were approaching and had caught up to a larger group of young adults. They informed us that they were part of a group traveling from New York State on a large commercial bus that had stopped to let them spend time in the Tetons. As we moved on, we came across several such groups most of which were making steady progress up the trail. One group, however, caught our interest because they were stopped, and many of them were leaning over the stream filling their drinking containers with raw stream water. Now in my reading, I had come to understand that giardia is very prevalent in Grand Teton National Park. In fact, one statistic that I had read stated that 100 percent of tested rodents were positive for giardia of a fairly virulent form. Here are these young people filling their containers with cold freshwater, which, I'm sure, would be refreshing to them but which was likely contaminated with giardia from the stream. After discussing this with my boys and deciding that I should probably warn them, I asked of the few nearest hikers if they were familiar with giardia. None of them had heard of the term.

I said, "Do you have a filter or chlorine tablets or anything to purify your water?" They replied that they did not. I did warn them of my knowledge of giardia in the area and for those who had not previously contaminated their water supply, I used my pump to provide can-clean filtered water for them to share. I also cautioned them as to the warning signs of giardia but spent the next fifteen minutes talking to my boys about how glad I was that we all were not part of that bus tour, having to experience waiting in line for restroom use for the next several days.

We hiked throughout the day to the top of Cascade Canyon and turned right at the top in a northerly direction toward the trail. Throughout the day, we had been circling around the backside of the Grand Teton Mountain. We saw many beautiful vistas and eventually came to the edge of Lake Solitude, which, disappointingly, was still completely frozen in late July. We backtracked to a campsite where we unpacked our tents, set them up, and fixed dinner. We enjoyed the beautiful views and the surrounding mountains but were quite tired from our day's hiking and turned in early. The night was chilly and was punctuated by a nice, cool dry wind.

The following morning, we awoke, broke camp, and began the trek southward back through the intersection at the top of Cascade Canyon and went on south to our next campsite. I noticed that my two boys had a lot of energy and spent most of their time scrambling over large boulders, climbing rock outcroppings, and hiking back and forth on short side trips. I, myself, was extremely tired after my hiking and carrying my pack. Now my plan was to have divided up the food so that each day, as we ate, everyone's pack would get a little lighter, mine included. My boys, however, had a different idea and had decided that morning to transfer several of the items they were carrying into my pack, instead. So my pack had gotten no lighter while there's had lost a few pounds each. My preparation and planning paid off well as we remained well-fed, fully hydrated, and warm while managing to attend all of our personal hygiene needs in accordance with park rules. This included packaging up and packing out all expelled urine and fecal material during our excursion.

The following morning, we awoke to find freshly fallen snow all over our tent and campground site. The weather warmed quickly and melted the snow, and other than a little slipperiness to the trail, the weather had no impact. We continued south through a pass and arrived at the entrance to Death Canyon, where we began our descent back into Teton Valley. A short time later, we ran across a group of hikers gathered over one of their party, who seemed to be having some difficulty. The individual in question was a female in her late teens who'd come up the canyon on a day hike but had become too faint to proceed, and her party members were trying to decide how best to get her down off the mountain. We had not seen a ranger since leaving the park headquarters two mornings before. I knew that they frequently hiked the trails and that one of them would be by in fairly short order, but my son-in-law and I were persuaded to try to effect the young woman's rescue while others in their party moved faster down the trail to obtain help. We took the time to provide oral fluid replacement for her, which didn't seem to make much of a change. I had no tools with which to take a blood pressure or do any other testing, but we did notice that she became faint each time she tried to stand upright. Fortunately, I was traveling with four people, myself included, who had received training as Boy Scouts. Additionally, I had taken a wilderness emergency course, which gave me some ideas toward implementing a transport device with which to help her down the canyon trail.

The six of us—my two boys, my son-in-law, myself, and two from the other hiker's party—all proceeded together down the trail with the patient while we awaited the arrival of the hoped-for park rangers. The remainder of the trip down was fairly uneventful except near the bottom of the trail to Death Canyon where the trail became shared by pack horses. There were no pack horses visible, but we had to step more carefully around piles of "road apples," as we picked our way along the trail. We finally arrived at the bottom of the trail, and there, in the flat area traversing the meadow, we found the long-awaited-for rangers. They took over the rescue procedure, used their radios to call in a helicopter, and proceeded to make arrangements to take the patient to the Jackson Hole Hospital. I never did see any specific injury and suspect that this patient had become dehydrated while hiking and combined with exhaustion from the exertion had simply ceded her ability to stay upright.

We completed our trail by looping north at the bottom of Death Canyon, finding our way back to park headquarters, checking out with the park rangers, informing them of our rescue of the hiker as well as the uninformed New York tourists and stopping for a well-deserved treat at the park supply shop. That was the best-tasting ice cream bar I can ever recall having eaten. I learned through the planning and implementation of this hike that I was, through my training and practice experience, reasonably prepared to intervene in most situations that could present themselves. Additionally, I became more aware of my abilities to intervene in those "sudden intimacy" moments that complete strangers might impose upon me, even during a vacation outing.

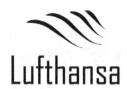

Lufthansa

I've had numerous opportunities to travel, and a couple of these trips have included being summoned for emergency assistance by the airline staff. This typically comes in the form of an announcement on the overhead paging system for any physician available to press the overhead call button adjacent to their seat. One such experience of this nature occurred during a transatlantic flight on a return trip from Greece. I had been visiting Greece while serving as an advisor to national fraternity organization and was serving as a mentor/advisor to a group of college students who had been invited on that trip. The overhead announcement was made by a thickly accented flight attendant who requested assistance from any physician aboard. I was seated in the middle section, aisle row of a large transatlantic aircraft. I was surrounded by students who had accompanied me on the journey and had shared many of the same experiences as I had. The young man sitting next to me looked at me quizzically and said, "Are you going to answer that?" I felt the earnestness of his question as well as my own obligation to serve and reached up and pressed the attendant call button.

The flight attendant quickly came down the aisle, reached up, and canceled my call button, leaned over, and quietly asked what kind of physician I was.

I told her, "Emergency medicine."

She replied quickly, "Great, come with me please." She took me to the front of the coach section of the aircraft, where a small group of people, perhaps three or four, were huddled.

One of the flight attendants was kneeling down over a middle-aged woman, who appeared pale but had her eyes closed and was listening but not speaking. The flight attendant told me that the woman had complained of dizziness and had requested assistance to the restroom, but upon helping her from her seat, had fainted. I introduced myself to the patient and the assembled staff, telling them that I was a practicing emergency physician and asking for them to obtain their first-aid kit.

As a part of my training, I had attended several meetings during which the contents and limitations of first-aid kits available to airline personnel were often discussed. I knew that some flights were better-equipped than others and might include simple medications, IV fluids, and perhaps even an onboard defibrillator. I had learned that there was great variability between the contents of first-aid kits within different airline corporations. I also had learned that most airlines subscribe to a formal service, based in the United States, available twenty-four hours a day, for fielding questions presented by flight attendant staff during flights when problems develop.

I took the patient's hand in mine and noted that it was cool and her hands were sweaty. She was able to open her eyes and respond to commands but didn't like to keep her eyes open. I quickly asked her medical history, including medications, allergies, and special historical medical problems. I asked where she was traveling from and what her destination would be and learned that she was from the country of India and had begun her journey approximately twelve to fourteen hours previously. She reported no serious medical problems, was taking no medications, and admitted no allergies. As a precaution, I inquired of her as to the possibility of pregnancy and was told that she was certain that she could not be pregnant.

Although we were total strangers, I carefully questioned her about any recent medical problems, conducting what is called a review of systems. This is something that I had memorized in order early on in my education and used frequently in evaluation of unknown problems. Essentially, it is a series of questions, such as Do you notice any problems? followed by a series of common problems. This would come in the form of a question, such as Any problems with dizziness, lightheadedness, vertigo, shortness of breath, chest pain? and so forth, covering all systems of the body in a head-to-toe direction. The reason for the head-to-toe direction is that I had the habit of actually looking at the patient as I asked the questions regarding each area, so as not to skip over any areas accidentally. Her systems review did not include any significant positives beyond the sudden onset of dizziness upon attempting to stand.

The first-aid kit arrived, and I found that it contained, among other items, a rather flimsy single-tube stethoscope. The area where the patient was lying down was a little noisy from the jet engine whine, but I decided to try to use the stethoscope anyway. The patient's pulse was very rapid when you listen through the stethoscope. It was very faint, and her breathing sounded normal to me. Her skin was warm but dry. She did not have the slow heart rate of sinus bradycardia, which is usually heard during fainting spells. Rather, she had the pale appearance and rapid heart rate suggestive of low blood pressure. Over the next several minutes of questioning, I learned that for the total duration of her journey from India to her present position approaching Detroit via the circumpolar route from Frankfurt, Germany, she had neither had anything to eat or drink. When asked about this, she rather embarrassingly related that she was afraid to eat or drink anything because she didn't want to have to get up and pee during the flight.

I then conducted a brief physical evaluation, including using the stethoscope, placing it external to her typical Hindu clothing to listen to her lungs and heart. The jet noise made this evaluation less than optimum, and I made note of my intention to try to encourage better quality stethoscopes for in-flight first-aid kits.

At about this time, the flight attendant returned from checking in with the captain, who had asked for an update and further asked, if in my estimation, we needed to divert to the nearest major airport, which was Detroit, or if we could proceed to Chicago's O'Hare, about forty-five minutes further.

The patient was stabilizing, had actually leaned upward a little during our conversation, and showed no further development of ill effects. I told the flight attendant the diversion of the flight would not be necessary, and we could proceed to our destination. I suggested that the captain contact the tower to have paramedics standing by to assist the patient off the airplane. Within the contents of the international first first-aid kit, I found a bag of sterile IV fluid as well as a variety of sizes of intravenous catheters and used the supplies to start a peripheral IV and begin the process of rehydrating this unfortunate patient.

I went back to my row and had my travel companions, except the assignment of gathering my book reader, made certain that my trash was cleaned up by the passing flight crew. I went back up to the front and found my patient recovering nicely with her head elevated and speaking to the flight crew attending her. I learned that the paramedics would meet us at the gate with a gurney to help retrieve the patient. Upon touchdown, I found myself in one of the rear-facing flight attendants' chairs seat-belted for safety during the landing. The flight attendants informed the passengers by overhead announcement that the medical emergency was resolving, but that they needed to stay in their seats until the patient was removed from the aircraft.

I greeted the Chicago paramedics upon their entry onto the airplane from the jetway. I told them my suspicions about the prolonged dehydration and the resulting effect on the patient's physiology during the long flight. They ran a quick EKG strip and assisted her off the airplane, down the jetway, and to the arriving passenger's reception area. I gave them one of my business cards, so they could identify me in the future and also asked for any updated information as it became available on the patient's condition.

I was allowed to go back on board, returned to my row, and met up with my travel companions. They all seemed quite impressed with my reports of success even though it wasn't the worst of medical problems that I had seen or treated. The flight attendants for Lufthansa promised to contact me with an updated condition of the patient, but I never did hear from them.

Overall, it was an enjoyable experience to have interacted with the flight crew on such a personal basis, to get to know so much about such a total stranger in so little time, and to contribute to the care and safety of a fellow passenger.

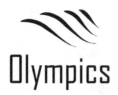

Olympics

When I first learned that Salt Lake City was to be the location hosting the 2002 Olympics, I initially paid little attention and didn't plan on participating whatsoever. In the two years leading up to all the competition, there was a lot of roadwork to be accomplished, and I saw this as just another nuisance with the potential for interference with travel and activities. Others in the larger cities to the south were actually planning on monetizing their Olympic experience by renting out their homes or other methods of cashing in on the large crowds anticipated. I first got interested in actually participating as a medical provider when some of my college hockey team players reported that they were signing up to volunteer in various capacities. We also learned, as a community, that we were having some Olympic teams use our newly completed ice arena as a venue for some pre-Olympic competitions and public display of figure skating. As the time approached, the medical provider for the Olympics was announced to be my employer, Intermountain Healthcare. This opened the door for me to serve as a volunteer medical provider, and I learned that one of my college team members was actually going to be serving in a supervisory capacity over portions of the hockey venue. This stimulated my interest, and I submitted my application and eventually was accepted to be a physician serving in the role of provider for visitor and spectator health services to be provided at the E Center.

Starting in fall of 2001, I began attending preparatory sessions of training for the upcoming Olympics. This was punctuated by the nation's experiencing the events of September 11, 2001. At the training sessions, each of us wondered how this would complicate our attendance and participation as Olympic providers. Eventually, as the training sessions progressed, we learned that Mitt Romney was going to be the CEO of the Olympic experience due to some financial irregularities that occurred in the lead up to the Olympics, including offering financial incentives to members of the International Olympic Committee in return for the choice of Salt Lake City as the venue. At our training sessions, we received specific instructions about being meticulous in any financial transactions regarding the Olympics and were cautioned against taking anything that might be construed as a bribe in regards to our participation.

At one of the training sessions in Salt Lake City, I was given several articles of clothing to be worn during my volunteer time at the Olympics. The outer garments were color-coded by category of service and included lavender for those involved in administrative roles, yellow for direct-venue service, and mine were bright-red indicating providers of medical services. We were required to attend training in international relations, customer service, and operation of our specific areas of responsibility. We were also issued tickets to the opening ceremony, access to the meal service area while on duty, and other amenities. I admit that I had some concerns about commuting the eighty minutes each way back and forth to Salt Lake City for my service opportunities, having concerns about traffic and weather.

As it turned out, my concerns were unfounded with the weather throughout my whole Olympic experience remaining nearly perfect, and traffic never being an issue. I was able to thoroughly enjoy my Olympic experience and came away with many new friends, fond memories, and even some tales to tell of a near international incident, which I almost caused.

Most of my Olympic experiences involved the direct provision of patient care to the visitors and staff of the E Center as mentioned. The first major event occurred during one of the early practice sessions, and a player from the West German team was struck in the face by a hockey puck, breaking several teeth and injuring his jaw. He was brought to the first-aid room by a trainer, but they rapidly found his team physician, who provided the majority of his care beyond simple first-aid. Most of what I treated involved rendering non-emergency evaluation and primary care for a variety of simple concerns. We handed out a lot of Band-Aids. Once the games actually started, I began to see event-related injuries that were unique to hockey. Overall, I watched fourteen games, including both men's and women's games, twelve of which were at the E Center and two of which were held in the Provo venue. Whenever the puck would leave the ice, I learned to anticipate someone in the crowded audience suffering an injury from being struck by the flying puck. Most often, this involved the head or neck area due to the fact that in the crowd these areas were exposed to injury.

One such patient was a young thirty-something male who was from Manhattan Island in New York City. He was employed by Visa Card services and was responsible for branding, which meant that he was responsible to see that their logo was always correctly displayed and within the color and visibility parameters specified by the parent company. It also meant that he had received very good seats to several of the hockey games throughout the week. At one game, when the puck left the ice, it struck his eyebrow causing a deep laceration of about an inch-and-a-half length. Now, in general, this is a common type of injury, which is received from some sort of blunt object striking the eyebrow and is commonly seen in children who are learning to walk. He came to the first-aid station on the second floor of the center holding a hand over his eyebrow and blood pouring between his fingers. He had not lost any consciousness, was not dizzy, nor showing any signs of concussion beyond the soft-tissue injury to the eyebrow. Being fairly young, he immediately expressed concerns over his injury asking if he needed to see a plastic surgeon. I discussed with him the location of the venue, about three to four miles from the nearest hospital with heavy evening traffic related to the business day as well as the Olympic games that were occurring that evening. I told him that it would be his choice as to whether or not to see a plastic surgeon but that we were fully capable of suturing that simple laceration but offered him the alternative of traveling to the nearest hospital to have the procedure completed. I warned him that if we transferred him, he would likely have a fifteen-to-twenty-minute drive to the hospital due to traffic, another fifteen-to-twenty-minute wait in the emergency department prior to service, followed by another fifteen-to-twenty-minute wait for the service to actually occur, followed by another twenty minutes or so to return back to the E Center, regain entry, and resume his seat. This would likely take him through the rest of the game and result in him missing any further game-watching experience that evening. I had a lot of confidence in my ability to provide a good plastic repair and thought that he would find the result acceptable if we were allowed to do it there at the center. With some hesitation, he agreed with the idea that he could always have the scar revised if in the future he found it excessive and unacceptable in appearance.

I cleaned the wound, further assessed for bony injuries, other injuries to the head and neck, and verified the absence of concussion. His eyebrow laceration was only slightly irregular along the edges, and the wound edges were easily matched up as a result of the jigsaw puzzle-like shape that resulted. As usual, I covered his face with a water-impermeable paper drape called an I Drape, which has a cutout in the center of it and covers most of the face, leaving the work area visible through the open hole. That meant that he was lying on his back, with only the injured eyebrow visible, and in this position, I could carry on a conversation unimpeded. I injected local anesthetic into the eyebrow, removing any further sensation and allowing me to begin work.

As we talked, I got to know more about him. He lived in downtown Manhattan, with a lifestyle that very nearly mirrored that of the Jerry Seinfeld character in the show of the same name. After college, he moved to Manhattan, got an apartment, and continued to live there as a single young male, enjoying all that Manhattan Island has to offer. Before long, the topic of September 11 came up. It turned out, he related, that he was in his office building on one of the upper levels when the first plane hit. Word quickly spread through his office building, resulting in many of his coworkers walking upward to the roof where they could see very clearly, just a few blocks away, the World Trade Center. He was standing there, looking toward the World Trade Center, when the second airliner came flying by just slightly above their building, tipped its wings, and flew into the second building of the World Trade Center and exploded. He related that, initially, he and the other bystanders were under the impression that it was just a serious accident, but then it became evident that this was likely intentional and that they were all in some danger due to their location. He related that they, over the next several minutes, received instructions to exit the building and did so running to the crowded subways along their escape route and eventually reaching a safe distance from the World Trade Center, prior to it falling to the ground. This amazing story was related to me while I sutured his eyebrow.

I finished suturing, placed a small compressive bandage over the eyebrow, gave him some aftercare instructions, and made arrangements for him to return to his seat. We agreed that he could go to any of the Olympic venues to have the sutures checked four or five days hence and have them removed if appropriate. That weekend, he was going to be attending a skiing event, again representing Visa, where he agreed to have the sutures checked. He asked me how much he owed for the sutures. I told him that I was there as a volunteer, that he didn't owe any money, and that in fact, I couldn't accept so much as a stick of gum from him due to the expressed concerns over the challenges presented by the initial bribery surrounding the acquiring of the 2002 Olympics. He returned back to his seat prior to the start of the third period, with an ice pack to place over his bandage and expressed gratitude for saving his Olympic experience. I thought that he had actually had a good result, and that he would show very little visible scar after healing.

A few days later, he returned to the first-aid station at the E Center. He stopped by to give me an updated report. He had gone to the ski venue first-aid station where the examining physician had asked him about his injury and was told all that had happened. The examining physician remarked to the patient that "Whoever sutured you did a very good job, and I don't think the scar will show." This made me feel very good, and as I examined him, I found that he was healing quite nicely, and although he was not particularly vain, it was nice to know that he would not have any untoward scarring as result of his experience. Once again, he asked me if he could pay me for the care that he received, and once again, I declined. During our conversation the previous week, I had told him that the university hockey team was due to travel to Manhattan in a couple of months for their national hockey tournament. He reminded me of that planned trip and asked if there was any way that he could meet me for dinner as a form of repayment for his care. I was elated that he was that happy with the outcome and told him that the Olympics would be over by that time and that I would not be under any further restrictions regarding accepting gratuities, and so I would try to make arrangements to meet him for dinner while in New York City. It turned out that I was able to make those plans, and we had dinner at a nice family restaurant just across the street from the hotel where John Lennon was killed. I traveled to that downtown location on the subway on the evening after my visit to the World Trade Center site, viewing the demolition that was ongoing and witnessing firsthand the broken glass windows, building damage, and other destruction still visible at that site. In all, it was a very touching ending to that Olympic experience.

A couple of other patients were noteworthy. One involved a young man who'd been taken to watch a hockey game by his father. They were in a crowd when, again, a puck left the ice, striking the young boy in the eyebrow, similar to the New Yorker. This patient received a significant laceration to the eyebrow, similar to the first, but had to suffer the indignity of having the puck quickly retrieved by the person sitting next to him in the crowd, denying him of the souvenir of a hard-earned Olympic puck. I got his laceration cleaned, numbed, and closed. Again, no other injuries noted, but I could tell that he had a lot of sadness over not being able to document his Olympic experience with the souvenir puck. I talked to the venue supervisor by radio, and by the time, we had the patient's eyebrow dressing ready to be applied, several very official Olympic administrators appeared in the doorway with a new souvenir puck from the 2002 Olympics. The patient related that his injury was now well-worth it because of the memories that he would have.

Other individuals treated during those Olympic days included an NBC cameramen whose job it was to control the steerable camera, which was focused on the goal at each end of the ice. This cameramen had become ill with symptoms of gastroenteritis, and I treated him with intravenous fluids, anti-nausea medication, and bedrest for several hours while he recuperated prior to his next hockey event. Another NBC staff member was a cook who worked for the NBC commissary that was set up at the venue. He had cut his finger on a sharp knife and required sutures for the injury. Finally, another puck injury was suffered by a middle-aged woman from Ohio who was the owner of a Hallmark retail store and was attending the Olympics as an invited sponsor. Each of these individuals provided a mutually shared Olympic experience and, in addition to the memories generated, resulted in the exchange of Olympic trading pins of various designs, which I saved into a collection of Olympic memories.

Now I should mention a little bit about the Olympic trading pins. This is a tradition that seems to accompany each Olympic celebration and dates back to an unknown amount of time. The Olympic trading pins are small painted enamel-coded metallic lapel pins that are created in shapes that represent elements of the local culture, current events, or other relevant shapes specific to that Olympics. For example, in the 2002 Winter Olympics, there were pins commemorating green Jell-O, 3.2 percent alcohol beer, Mormon missionaries on bicycles, as well as the oven mittens representing the NBC commissary, and several corporate logos. It seemed everyone was trying to find the green Jell-O pin, but my favorite pin was the one given out by the Utah Highway Patrol, which included red-and-blue flashing LED lights attached to a police cruiser, shaped pin that was powered by a small hearing aid battery. I would stop by a store on my morning trip to Salt Lake City to the E Center and shop for the newest designs that I could find. Another pin that I saw but was impossible to obtain was the one given out by the Secret Service, which consisted of a small black diamond shape. This identified various elements of the security detail and was present on the lapels of every Secret Service agent when VP Cheney came to the E Center to watch a hockey game. The pin that I gave out was a small enamel-colored hockey-skate-shaped pin that became my trademark for trading pins in the hallway in between events. During these times, you could always wander the halls of the venue and find people trading pins informally. The tradition as it was expressed in 2002 was that if a pin was visible, it was tradable and could be requested, but that you always got another pin in return. A few months after the Olympics, I had occasion to travel to Germany to the village of Garmisch-Partenkirchen, which was the site of the 1932 Olympics just prior to World War II. In one of the souvenir stores in that village, there were still pins available from that era. Upon my return home from Germany, I sent a package to the shopkeeper that included a dozen or so of the more modern Olympic version, and this gift was very warmly received by the shop owner.

My favorite Olympic experience, however, was one that I'd already hinted at previously. I nearly started an international incident toward the end of the Olympic competition. The United States team had won its initial competitions and was slated to play the semifinal game against the Russian competitors. There had been a lot of publicity in the run-up to the game with the result that the Russian team accused the US team of spying on its practices and, due to the suspicion of cheating, asked for the practices to be closed to the public. Now on the date of the scheduled practice sessions, the practices were indeed closed, with no one allowed in the area of the E Center ice arena, including vendors, news reporters, photographers, or other observers. The only individuals allowed in the area of the ice were the Zamboni driver and net crew in addition to the first-aid team, which that day were scheduled to be me and two paramedics. Practices were ninety minutes in length; after which, the ice was cleared. The Zamboni was run out to cut the ice, and the nets were replaced, following which, the other team would take the ice for practice. The US team completed their practice uneventfully with no injuries or significant events.

The Russian team came on to the ice, and while they practiced, I sat and idly chatted with the paramedics. I really didn't see anything special and witnessed no injuries during the practice. Now if I had seen any injuries, it was important to know that each of the teams had their own professional sports medicine staff accompanying them and certainly would've been capable of taking care of any injuries that resulted during the practice. However, the Olympic regulations required the presence of first responders in the first-aid provider on-site at the venue during the course of the practice. The three of us sat at the side of the arena, just inside the glass. For the duration of the practice, we were situated at the north end of the E Center ice arena so that we could watch the visiting goalie go through his workout. He was actively involved in an exercise where the coach would repeatedly fire the puck just outside of his reach requiring that he skate over outside of the net, clear the puck, and return back into the net before the second shot could be taken at him. The coach was actually pretty good at getting the puck past him just out of his reach and stretching his abilities to retrieve the loose puck. The goalie was getting quite tired by this time in the practice, and I think was a little short-tempered a few times when the coach shot the puck at him. Very soon, the player peeled off his helmet, threw it down on the ice, shouted something in Russian to the coach, and skated away a few strides before returning to the net and assuming his defensive position. A few shots later, the coach again put a puck just outside the reach of the goalie, resulting in the goalie having to stretch out and extend his length to its extreme. The second time, he peeled off his helmet, threw it down, causing it to skitter across the ice; after which, the goalie started to skate down the ice alone. I looked around and saw that the practice was over, and it was just the goalie and the coach remaining on the ice. Now remember the E Center was closed for this practice. No other individuals were in the arena, just the goalie coach, the goalie, and the three medical staff.

What I saw was the perfect Kodak moment. With the empty E Center as a background, the goalie coach skated down toward the center of the ice, following the goalie. There were just the two of them in the completely empty E Center with the coach placing his arm around the shoulder of the goalie, reassuring him and calming him after he lost his temper. Without thinking about it, I reached down, and next to me on the seat, pulled up my camera and snapped a picture. I had forgotten that the practice was closed to photography, and I'd forgotten to turn off my flash, and there in the empty E Center saw the bright flash light up the venue of the two Russian team members. Both the goalie coach and the goalie immediately turned and started skating toward us sitting in the first row. Now the two paramedics on either side of me immediately stood and bolted up the stairs and out the doors, leaving me all alone to face their wrath. I began to quickly plan my response, not understanding any Russian whatsoever, and wondering how I would be able to explain away the bright flash when no photography was allowed during that practice session. I quickly visualized the international incident that would result from my spying on a closed practice in that manner. My heart began to pound as they skated closer and closer, but I realized that there was a large glass wall between us and while they could see me, they were not going to be able to physically strike me. I thought about how to overcome my language skill lack, and I thought that if I gestured that I was sorry, especially if I touched my hand to my chest in a sign of sincerity, they might understand my regret. It was a digital camera, and so I didn't have any film to pull out and expose to the light to surrender the photo. Instead I stood, faced the two of them as they skated up to the edge of the ice, and mouthed the words "I'm very sorry."

The goalie bent forward, and using his goalie stick, wrapped the tip of the stick on the ice surface against a loose puck that was lying on the ice after the practice session, and skillfully flipped the puck over the glass wall to me, where I caught it in my hand. I smiled at both the player and the coach. I later learned that this goalie was in everyday life a Russian immigrant who played for the Chicago Blackhawk professional hockey team and probably understood English completely and could've communicated fully about the situation. Regardless, I still have that hockey puck, obtained from that player during that Olympic practice. I also still have the photograph, and it turned out great!

That event stood out so prominently in my mind that I barely remembered the championship game that year against Canada and the resulting celebration.

Sports Medicine Experience

My third career, after family medicine and spending considerable time in emergency medicine, involved the practice of sports medicine. These three careers overlapped quite a bit, with my sports medicine career actually beginning soon after starting my practice in Tremonton. I had the good fortune to make the acquaintance of the brand-new local high school football coach that moved to town about the same time I did and shared my backyard fence. My wife and I went over and introduced ourselves to him and his wife and brought them a plate of cookies. I learned that he was the new football coach at Bear River High School and he learned that I was a new physician in the community. Before we finished our conversation, he asked me if I followed any of the teams in the area, and I replied that I did not, and he asked if I'd be willing to come and spend some time on his sideline and help them with the medical care of his team. Thus began a long and enjoyable association that spanned multiple coaches, multiple teams, and multiple schools. At one point in time, I even considered taking the examination and becoming certified in the practice of sports medicine but chose not to for a couple of reasons. First, there was a short window of time available for family physicians to "grandfather in" to certification in sports medicine, and I wasn't sure that I could complete the examination process within the deadline, and the second reason was that it would have cost quite a bit to take the examination and would not have changed my income at all at the time I was making a decision.

My interest in sports medicine was stimulated further by my involvement in the practice of providing care to teams in the area augmented by frequent consultation with an outstanding orthopedic surgeon, who also dedicated a lot of his practice to sports medicine.

Through frequent consultations, participation in conferences, and actual practice of sideline medicine, I gained sufficient experience to reach a level of expertise that allowed me access to high school and then college teams. As a result of this series of experiences, I had the opportunity to see a lot of games, participate in the care of many student athletes, attend the 2002 Olympics (as I've previously mentioned), and to provide care for some very interesting sports injuries. On some weeks, between teams that I was providing care for or coaching, it was my privilege to watch as many as nine competitive games in one weekend. I found that, by far, providing care for student athletes left me feeling very young for a very long time.

Over the years, there had been many situations, both emergent and nonemergent, that came to my attention in the practice of sports medicine. During the course of this time, I provided care for sports teams involving football, soccer, volleyball, gymnastics, hockey, rugby, lacrosse, and wrestling. What I learned was that it really didn't matter whether you were competing for a medal, an award, or just the final score. When gravity won, results were often the same. Sports medicine also gave me many opportunities to travel as the team physician. These experiences were both good and bad. Some of the *good* times involved attending and traveling to such exotic locations as the University of Alabama, where I looked into the stands before the game and saw way far up in the southeast corner of the Alabama Stadium very back row of seats in the worst position possible within that stadium contain the seat back chair of the seat's owner. How would it be? I also had the not-so-good opportunity of spending thirty consecutive hours on a bus traveling through winter snow back from Southern California through Donner Pass. That was a trip that normally takes about fourteen hours. As a member of the medical team providing care for the Utah State Aggies, I won four bowl rings!

One of my most memorable experiences involved the Utah State Hockey team while playing the team from Denver University at our local ice sheet. Midway through the second period, I saw a collision between one of our players and a visitor when the visitor got hard checked into the glass surrounding the ice. This collision rattled the glass and resulted in the collapse of the Denver player as the two skated apart. As the visiting team's physician, I had responsibility to provide first response/first aid to the visiting team if they did not have a trainer present. A lot of times, this policy led to raised eyebrows as I walked into the visitors' locker room with my logo-bearing jacket clearly visible. Opposing teams were, in general, happy to see me and fully accepting of my advice. In this situation, Denver University had a team trainer, who headed out to check on the player who had remained prone on the ice beyond the time that I would've expected him to require to return to upright position. When players went down, I usually started to leave my position on the team bench because, at the very least, I would probably have to check them when they returned to their team box. In this case, however, I saw that the player was lying motionless on the ice surface.

Because the ice was extremely slippery and I didn't wear skates in the coaches' box, I had the habit of relying on my own trainer to help support me (with balance) as I scooted across the ice with shuffling feet. It was an acquired ability to be able to walk on a slick ice sheet without skates or special shoe coverings. As I made my way across the ice to where the collision had occurred, I noticed that the down player was still not moving, which, while an ominous sign, is most often related to the desire by the opposing player to have the instigator of the collision called for a penalty. In this situation, however, the injury that had occurred was due to sufficient velocity and power that it was legitimate.

I shuffled over, knelt down on the surface of the ice, and told the player, "Don't move."

He responded, "Don't worry, I can't!"

This made my heart start to beat rapidly, and I immediately reached to support his head and neck to prevent any sudden movement. The visiting trainer witnessed this and immediately sprang into action, checking his player's grip strength, shoulder strength, and movement in the lower extremities. The two of us determined that, while the patient was awake, he was indeed lacking sensation to his arms, legs, and lower back. He reported that he had felt a sudden "electric shock" sensation at the time of the impact. He was not having difficulty breathing and remained able to speak clearly, impaired only by the presence of his helmet chinstrap. Again, due to the high-energy mechanism of injury and the fact that he was not recovering any movement, I signaled, by a prearranged hand signal that we used at the ice arena, to the sheriff's deputy that attended each of the home games. I held my right hand to my ear, phone-like, and mouthed "Call 911." He nodded in acknowledgment of the message. Over the next several minutes, the remaining members of the team skated around their home benches, giving us space to work. The young man's father, who was in the visitors' gallery from Colorado, appeared at the side of his son and was informed as to the nature of the suspected injury.

My examination showed no step off the cervical spine, but there was significant tenderness at the base of the neck beneath the helmet.

Hockey helmets are different from football helmets in that they are much more loosely fitting, are held in place solely by a loose-fitting chinstrap, and don't cause as much displacement of the cervical spine if left in place. Likewise, hockey shoulder pads are much thinner and do not cause and cure displacement of the neck if left in place. The shoulder pads provide additional insulation and distance from the underlying frigid ice. It was therefore our policy in such situations as this, to leave the shoulder pad and helmet in place until the neck was fully stabilized. After about six or seven minutes, the paramedics arrived at the ice sheet, bringing the ambulance gurney carefully across the ice.

We used a carefully coordinated team approach to maintain in-line stability of the patient's cervical spine during the lifting, repositioning, and transporting of the victim. This is actually something I practiced with their own training team as well as rehearsed myself on several occasions. I checked the neurologic function of the upper extremities, lower extremities, and low back in addition to rechecking the patient's level of consciousness at several intervals. Prior to the arrival of the paramedics, I also called the hospital emergency department, forewarning them of the potential cervical spine injury with neurological loss.

While the paramedics were transporting the injured player, I transported his father in my private vehicle to the emergency department and arrived at about the same time as the patient was being transferred into his bed in the emergency department. By that time, he had noticed the return of a small amount of sensation in his hands and feet, which was a very good sign, indeed. He had the usual stabilization (IV, vitals, pain medication, as well as intravenous steroids for his suspected cord injury). An immediate CT scan of his upper spine was obtained and showed the presence of a C2 fracture of his spine. This fracture was the same as that suffered by the actor Christopher Reeve, *Superman* of movie fame.

I reviewed the findings of his CT scan with the physician on duty in the ER as well as with the patient's father. A quick recheck of his neurologic status showed that he was regaining more sensation into his upper extremities and could now feel his lower extremities, which was reassuring and meant that his initial "electric shock" sensation was probably due to some temporary cord pressure and not due to transection. The patient was further stabilized and flown by air ambulance to the waiting neurosurgeon at the Salt Lake City level 1 trauma center, where he underwent immediate surgery, which placed some screws in his upper cervical spine to stabilize the bony prominence of the C-2 axis. This two-bone pairing of vertebrae in the upper spine served as both the pin and ring upon which the doughnut of the C1 vertebrae sits and allows it to rotate freely, limited only by the ligaments that allow rotation of the head up on the neck. Thus stabilized, the patient was able to return home and return to the University of Denver a few weeks later but did not return to skating or hockey playing.

I believe the care that this young man received from the trainers, paramedics, and emergency physicians served to protect his neurologic function and prevent any further injury or loss. I wrote a letter to Denver University complimenting this trainer on his abilities and delivery of care to that player at that event. This certainly could have resulted in catastrophic loss for an otherwise healthy young man in the prime of his life.

While nothing quite so exciting as the neck injury had occurred before, or since, I had many opportunities to provide care to other injured players along the way. These injuries consisted of a lot of lacerations, contusions, sprains, ligament injuries, dislocations, and other assorted related injuries. I got pretty adept at placing sutures in areas of poor lighting, cold ambient temperature, and other extreme conditions. I think one measure of success was when you could repair a laceration to an injured referee's earlobe and do it within the ten-minute break between periods during the competition. Over the next couple of seasons, I saw the same referee at several consecutive games, and he was very happy with the outcome and invisible scar.

Most of these experiences were, by far, positive ones. The only time I regretted my close association with a hockey team involved a road trip to the national tournament being held at Rutgers University in New Jersey. Not exactly a sports-related injury, but the team decided they would go downtown after their last game of the tournament to let off steam and get some Philly steak sandwiches. As they departed, I warned them to be back in the hotel prior to the cabs closing down because we had an early flight the next day, and I wanted some sleep prior to returning the rental vehicles to the airport checkout location. Sure enough, at about 1:00 a.m., my phone rang, and I responded sleepily, "I told you not to call" and hung up immediately. Thirty seconds or so later, the phone rang a second time, and a second time, I said, "I told you not to call," and hung up again.

They called the third time, just a few moments later, and before I could say anything, I heard, "Doc, don't hang up. This is our last quarter."

I sleepily asked what they wanted, and they said, "We need a ride. All the cabs have stopped."

I was more awake now, so I said, "Walk," in my firmest voice.

The voice on the other end of the line sheepishly replied, "Some of us can't walk."

I spent the next half hour searching and found them walking in a crooked line down the middle of the street. I picked them up, then spent the hour after that searching for a twenty-four-hour carwash to clean up the emesis that had occurred on the quick return trip to the hotel. I got that all cleaned up and returned the van with the still-wet carpet to the airport in time to make the return flight. While I still consented to travel with the team on future trips, I did not again have to serve in the babysitting capacity.

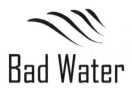

Bad Water

One of the not-so-funny episodes that occurred as a result of my involvement with sports medicine came about one late summer as the team was preparing for the upcoming season. It was their habit to have an end-of-summer camp wherein they meet at a remote location for conditioning, training, and development of team connections. This particular year, a local rancher had offered the use of his property for the team to visit and go through their workout plans in quiet seclusion. The temperatures were still quite warm during the day and careful attention had to be paid to the potential for dehydration.

After a particularly intense workout, which involved a lot of running, the team was released as a group for rest and rehydration. What happened after that practice was related to me later that day by the coach, who contacted me in anticipation of some expected complications. The team was dismissed by the coaching staff, being hot and thirsty. They all lined up at a coiled garden hose that was located on the property. The whole team took their turn drinking from the garden hose one by one. It was after nearly all the team had slaked their thirst that the rancher stopped by and, with a surprised look on his face, informed the group that the hydrant from which they were drinking was secondary water.

Now in Utah, irrigation is very common, it being a desert environment. *Secondary water* is a term used for water that is conveyed via an open ditch and is used for irrigation purposes and is not generally potable. It is usually designated by the presence of a red-painted handle on the spigot or faucet to the hose connection. Many of the boys knew this method of designating secondary water but had not paid attention to the presence of this warning sign.

The source for the water in this instance was a gravity-fed line that started in an irrigation canal a couple of hundred yards upstream. Also located upstream were cattle pastures, poultry pens, and a variety of other animal enclosures. When the coaching staff realized that the whole team had been exposed to this secondary water, they called me to see what steps they should take. I immediately called the health department and discussed the situation with them in an effort to learn what common water-borne illnesses were present in this area. I immediately made arrangements to have a team meeting that night with the parents and players to give the best information.

We met together that evening at the local high school in a meeting that was attended by parents, players, and coaches. I described them the symptoms that might develop, which included nausea, vomiting, and of course, diarrhea. I prepared them for the potential outbreak of such conditions as campylobacter, pathogenic E. coli, giardia, salmonella, and any other conditions that I could think of. The problem was that it was going to take an incubation of between three days and two weeks for any of these conditions to show themselves. In the meantime, we could only really wait on the developing situation. The team was also facing the prospect of starting their first game in two weeks with a significant portion of their team disabled.

This was my first experience in large-scale public health, but it taught me many valuable lessons. I learned that not everyone who was exposed to communicable disease of this nature would develop it. Furthermore, I learned that enteric bacteria only reproduce at a set rate, and there was nothing that one can do or say that would speed the process and return the culture results more quickly. Finally, I learned that, no matter how well-connected you were, you would need to wait for the culture results along with everyone else. The father of one of the team members couldn't understand why the health department was recommending on basing antibiotic treatment on actual culture results rather than prophylactic treatment and so pressured the school administration and coaching staff with threats of calling the governor in order to obtain the culture results more quickly. As it turned out, it didn't matter whether you know the governor or not, bacteria only reproduce at a set rate, can't be sped up, and allow the culture results to be read only after a significant incubation interval.

We did end up having a dozen or so positive cultures, which were treated with simple antibiotics and resolved completely. The team ended up playing the first game, mostly at full strength, and went on to do well that season. I became well-acquainted with the health department and was, in no small part due to my experiences here, invited to join the local area board of health.

One of the more colorful characters that I had the pleasure of associating with was the head athletic trainer at the university. He was a Hall of Fame recipient, had worked at the Armed Forces Academy at West Point, and was responsible for my learning the ins and outs of a lot of sports medicine as practiced at the university level. He was plainspoken, and most often, you knew where you stood with him. He had a very pragmatic approach to sports medicine, and we developed a good working relationship.

He appreciated my abilities and primary care training, stating on more than one occasion, "What I need is a family doctor, and when I need an orthopedic surgeon, I will rent one." He was also the source for the bits of wisdom known as the four principles of management, which I plagiarized.

The four principles of management are "I can do that;" "I have done that before;" "I could do it again;" and "But if I need to, I won't need you!"

It was on the recommendation of this athletic trainer that I began teaching, with other members of the physical education department, a graduate-level class in sports medicine for athletic trainers. The payoff for teaching this class was, in addition to reestablishing a teacher-student relationship, was learning to get up early in the morning in order to be at class before going to my regular job that began at eight o'clock each morning. It was a challenge, however, to always prepare myself in such a way as to know more than the students whom I was teaching. This allowed me to review much of the curriculum of sports medicine.

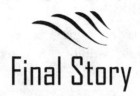

Final Story

Where does that bring us? As I mentioned at the beginning, medicine enables the practitioner to develop rapid and deep "sudden intimacies" with many of those around us, especially patients. The true basis of this relationship stemmed from the authority granted to practicing physicians by the patient. It had been amazing, through my career, to witness firsthand the depth of some of these enabled intimacies. The secrets and deep, inner thoughts that were shared within this work should, by no means, be taken lightly. I had been privileged to share in the process of birth, physical affliction, joy, pleasure, pain, and ultimately, death. Along the way, I had been personally inspired and uplifted by those who had been open with their histories and experiences. I had also been, at times, saddened and depressed by the life experiences of those around me.

Medicine is an amazing profession, which allows those with the special privilege of its practice to sometimes view the inner workings of this world. I have been always amazed at how much "in the know" that these experiences have allowed me to become. Medicine is a profession that, if practiced as it should be practiced, requires much from the provider and grants much in the form of rewards. I have appreciated greatly the trust placed within me through this great experience.

Just near my sixty-fifth birthday, I suffered, without any forewarning, a serious stroke. This event essentially ended my career in family, emergency, and sports medicine. With my limited abilities remaining, I wanted to share this collection of amazing experiences and, particularly, the notion of "sudden intimacies" as they relate to the learning and practice of medicine.

I hope that you have enjoyed the experiences as much as I have enjoyed relating them.

About the Author

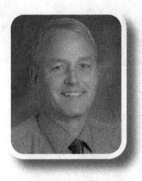

Dr. Jim Davis MD was born in Washington, Iowa. He did his undergraduate schooling at Monmouth College in Monmouth, Illinois, and medical school at the University of Iowa in Iowa City, Iowa. He and his wife, Cathy, have five children and twenty grandchildren. Prior to his retirement in 2017, he enjoyed hiking, traveling, woodworking, welding, and he was an avid gardener. He now resides in Utah, enjoying family, reading, and biking the trails of southern Utah.

CPSIA information can be obtained
at www.ICGtesting.com
Printed in the USA
JSHW030942140221
11848JS00004B/2

9 781662 415296